Copyright © 2025 by Hemant Patel. All Rights Reserved.

No part of this book may be copied, reproduced, stored in a retrieval system, or transmitted in any form or by any means—electronic, mechanical, photocopying, recording, or otherwise—without prior written permission from the author or publisher, except for brief quotations in reviews or articles, or as permitted by applicable copyright laws.

Disclaimer Notice:

This book is intended for informational and educational purposes only. All effort has been executed to present accurate, up to date, and reliable, complete information. The author and publisher disclaim any liability for the misuse or misinterpretation of the information contained herein. The content does not constitute medical, legal, or professional advice. Readers acknowledge that the author is not engaging in the rendering of legal, financial, medical or professional advice. The content within this book has been derived from various sources.

Readers should consult relevant professionals before making any decisions based on the material.

All trademarks, product names, and company names mentioned in this book are the property of their respective owners.

By reading this document, the reader agrees that under no circumstances is the author responsible for any losses, direct or indirect, which are incurred as a result of the use of the information contained within this document, including, but not limited to, — errors, omissions, or inaccuracies.

Legal Notice:

This book is copyright protected. This book is only for personal use. You cannot amend, distribute, sell, use, quote or paraphrase any part, or the content within this book, without the consent of the author or publisher.

For permissions, inquiries, or licensing requests, please contact:

hemant.AIGuide@selfcarenation.co.uk

DISCLAIMER

Disclaimer

While all the nutrients and dietary changes referred to in this book have been proven safe, those seeking help for specific medical conditions are advised to consult a qualified clinical nutritionist, doctor, or equivalent health professional. The recommendations provided in this book are intended solely for educational and informational purposes and should not be taken as medical advice. Neither the authors nor the publisher accept liability for readers who choose to self-prescribe.

All medicines and supplements should be kept out of reach of infants and young children.

To my beloved parents

To my late mother, whose love and healing lived in every vegetarian and non-vegetarian meal,
and to my father, whose life in yoga and thirst for knowledge continue to inspire mine.
With deep gratitude and love, always.

To my beloved family, especially the grandchildren

Thank you for your love and support, and especially for bearing with me while I hid away in my little office to research and write this book.
Through the demands of public life and the quiet hours of writing, your laughter, patience, and presence reminded me daily of what truly matters.

To my profession of pharmacy

Thank you for the lifelong opportunity to serve, to learn,
and to witness the power of science and compassion working hand in hand.
It has been both a calling and a privilege to walk alongside those seeking healing.

To my country, the United Kingdom, that gave us home, security and prosperity

Thank you for the freedom to dream, the safety to grow, and the chance to contribute -
all made possible by the enduring values upheld by King and country.
May this book be one small way of giving back to the nation that gave so much.

To my friends

Thank you for standing by me through the challenges of public life and leadership.
Your support during testing times has been a quiet pillar of strength, and I remain deeply grateful.

CONTENTS

Fullpage image	VI
Introduction	1
1. Understanding Chronic Inflammation	7
2. The Hidden Pandemic – How Medications Are Fueling Nutrient Deficiencies and Inflammation	19
3. Food is Medicine	30
4. Movement is Medicine	39
5. Spices Are Medicine	47
6. Mental Health & Whole-Body Well-Being	55
7. Holistic Health & Behavior Change	69
8. Addressing Common Objections	78
9. Practical Solutions for Busy Lifestyles	86
10. Exploring the World through Food – A Culinary Journey	94
11. Science-Backed Approaches to Healing and Wellness	104
12. Digital, Community and Global Engagement	111
Conclusion	119
Fullpage image	123
Glossary and References	124

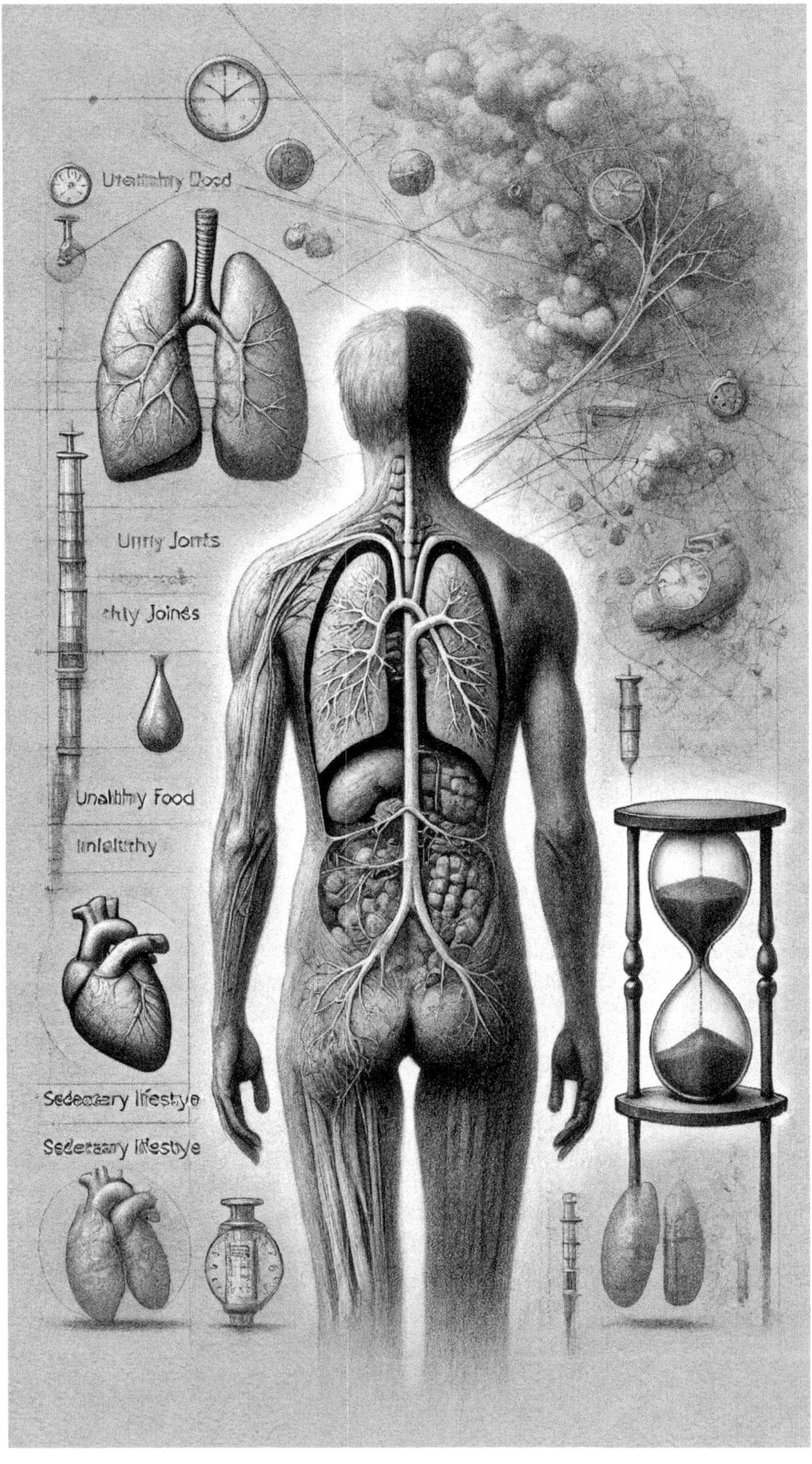

INTRODUCTION
Reverse Chronic Inflammation

In the spring of 2020, I found myself in a fight for my life. COVID-19 hit me hard, stripping away my strength, causing rapid weight loss and extreme weakness, and leaving me unable to walk unaided. Every breath felt like a battle. As I lay in bed, struggling to do what had once been effortless, I was confronted with a terrifying reality - uncertainty, fear, and the realization that my future was no longer in my control. My family surrounded me, offering love and support, but I could see the worry in their eyes. I re-read my will at my weakest, questioning whether I would survive to see the future I had worked so hard to build.

The experience changed me. It didn't just affect my body – it reshaped my entire understanding of health. But with time, determination, and the right support, I found hope. And I realized something powerful: we are not powerless in the face of illness. We can rebuild and reclaim our health by understanding our bodies and making the right choices. This empowerment, this understanding, is the key to taking control of our health and feeling confident in our ability to manage it.

As a pharmacist, a recognized leader in pharmacy, a champion of public health, and a passionate advocate for tackling health inequalities, I have spent my career working to improve healthcare – not just through medicine but by addressing the root causes of disease. My experience with COVID-19 reinforced something I have always believed: prevention is just as important as treatment. As I recovered, I asked more profound questions: Why do some people struggle to recover while others bounce back? What makes us more vulnerable to illness in the first place? This turning point led me to investigate the hidden force behind so many chronic conditions – inflammation – and, more importantly, how we can control it.

Why This Book Matters

As a former President of the Royal Pharmaceutical Society of Great Britain and now a dedicated health coach, I have spent my career advocating for preventive healthcare. My background in pharmacy and my commitment to reducing health inequalities have reinforced one clear truth: we cannot merely treat illnesses; we must address their root causes. It is essential to empower individuals, families, and communities with the knowledge to take charge of their health. This community support, this shared journey towards better health, is vital and can make a significant difference in our health management.

This book is not just about theory. It's a practical roadmap designed to help you fight inflammation with simple, evidence-based strategies that seamlessly fit into your daily life. It empowers you to take control of your health in realistic, sustainable, and scientifically backed ways. These strategies are not daunting or difficult; they are manageable and can be integrated into your life with ease, giving you the reassurance that you can make a positive change for your health.

The Growing Burden of Chronic Inflammation

Chronic inflammation is the silent force behind diseases like diabetes, heart disease, arthritis, certain cancers, and even depression. The current medical model is often reactive, focusing on symptom management rather than prevention. This leads to an over-reliance on medications - many of which are necessary but can also contribute to a cycle where long-term drug use becomes the norm. The consequences go beyond side effects; some medications can deplete essential nutrients, a lesser-known issue called drug–induced nutrient deficiency (DIND), which can further fuel inflammation and slow recovery.

The COVID-19 pandemic further highlighted the devastating effects of unchecked inflammation. Millions of people continue to suffer from post-COVID syndrome (long COVID), dealing with relentless fatigue, brain fog, breathlessness, and chronic pain. Research now points to low-grade, persistent inflammation as a key driver of these symptoms, interfering with immune regulation, metabolism, and neurological function. But there's hope. Targeted lifestyle interventions – like an anti–inflammatory diet, movement adapted to individual capacity and stress management – are emerging as powerful tools for recovery. Whole, nutrient-rich foods, such as those in the Mediterranean diet, have been linked to improved immune resilience in long COVID sufferers. Thoughtfully paced physical activity can also help rebuild strength, but overexertion can worsen symptoms for those experiencing post-exertional malaise (PEM), making a personalized approach essential.

I wasn't sure if I'd regain my strength at my lowest point, and my fear of permanent damage was confirmed. But I learned that healing is possible – not just for those recovering from COVID-19 but for anyone battling chronic inflammation. The key lies in addressing the root causes, rebuilding resilience, and restoring control of our health.

Breaking the Cycle: Food, Movement, and Resilience

Recent research has shed light on the complex relationship between chronic inflammation (the body's prolonged immune response), hyperinsulinemia (abnormally high insulin levels), and oxidative stress (cell damage caused by an imbalance between free radicals and antioxidants). Together, these processes can fuel a vicious cycle that worsens chronic disease. The good news? This cycle can be broken with the right lifestyle choices: i) Ditch ultra-processed foods that promote oxidative stress and inflammation ii) Embrace nutrient-rich, whole foods packed with antioxidants and anti-inflammatory compounds iii) Stay active – movement is a powerful tool for reducing insulin resistance and inflammation.

The Role of Food Literacy

The challenges faced by the Margate food bank, where fresh vegetables often go untouched, highlight a significant barrier to better health – food illiteracy. Many younger individuals lack basic cooking skills, opting for processed convenience foods over nutritious options. This not only leads to wasted food but also fuels the rise of chronic inflammation and nutrient deficiencies.

Dr. Fiona Lavelle, a lecturer in Nutritional Sciences at King's College London, emphasizes the critical role of food literacy in building a healthy society. She advocates for early culinary education, suggesting that even toddlers can begin learning basic food preparation skills. Individuals can shift their dietary habits by overcoming the fear of handling raw ingredients and building confidence in cooking, ultimately improving long-term health outcomes. In many communities, food literacy programs are being used to combat the rise in chronic diseases, reinforcing the idea that food is not just a means of survival but a powerful tool for health and well-being.

Inspiring Community Health Initiatives

Around the world, communities are proving that health isn't just about personal choices – it's about our environment. Inspired by the Blue Zones – places where people live longer, healthier lives – several cities and towns have implemented grassroots health initiatives. For example, in Kona, Hawaii, residents have embraced a plant-forward diet, daily physical activity, and strong social connections to support longevity and well-being. Similarly, in Copenhagen, Denmark, the city's bike-friendly infrastructure, active lifestyles, and a strong sense of community have increased residents' health and happiness. These initiatives demonstrate that when people come together with a shared vision, they can create lasting, transformative changes for future generations.

Your Journey to Better Health Starts Here

"Food is Medicine" and "Movement is Medicine" are more than catchy phrases - they are fundamental truths. Eating, moving, and managing stress directly influence inflammation and overall health. This book will guide you through the profound impact of nutrition, movement, and even spices on your body, showing you how to harness these tools to prevent and reverse chronic inflammation. Whether you're struggling with chronic pain, long COVID, or want to optimize your well-being, this book is for you. It takes a holistic approach, recognizing that health isn't just about avoiding disease but thriving at every stage of life.

What Makes This Book Different?

This book is not just about information - it's about action. Drawing from my professional expertise and personal journey, I aim to make health enhancement accessible, realistic, and sustainable. By adopting the principles in this book, you can reclaim your health, empower your family, and contribute to a movement that reduces the burden on our healthcare system. Your journey starts now, and I'm honored to walk this path with you.

Your Anti-Inflammatory Journey: One Step at a Time

A journey of a thousand miles doesn't begin with a leap - it begins with a single, deliberate step.

This is your space to take those steps. After each chapter, take a moment to pause, reflect, and decide on one small change you're ready to make. Use the prompts below to set clear, achievable goals - not sweeping resolutions, but realistic, meaningful actions that fit your life. Let this be how you ensure the investment you've made - in this book and in your time - truly pays off.

The best goals are SMART: Specific | Measurable | Achievable | Relevant | Time-bound

Think of it as building momentum, chapter by chapter. You're not trying to overhaul your entire life overnight - just keep moving forward, one intentional choice at a time.

Chapter commitment	Describe your
Introduction	I will...
Chapter 1: Understanding Chronic Inflammation	I will...
Chapter 2: The Hidden Pandemic	I will...
Chapter 3: Food is Medicine	I will...
Chapter 4: Movement is Medicine	I will...
Chapter 5: Spices Are Medicine	I will...
Chapter 6: Mental Health & Whole-Body Well-Being	I will...
Chapter 7: Holistic Health & Behavior Change	I will...
Chapter 8: Addressing Common Objections	I will...
Chapter 9: Practical Solutions for Busy Lifestyles	I will...
Chapter 10: Exploring the World through Food	I will...
Chapter 11: Science-Backed Approaches	I will...
Chapter 12: Digital, Community	I will...

Keep this page visible - revisit it after reading each chapter or as often as you like. It's your reminder that progress is possible, and it starts with just one thing.

When You've Completed All 12 Actions

Congratulations - you've done far more than just read. You've turned knowledge into momentum, and momentum into meaningful change.

Take a moment now to reflect on the journey. This isn't the end - it's the foundation of a healthier future that you've already started building, one choice at a time. Commit to keeping these habits alive, adjusting them as you grow. And if you've missed a step along the way? No shame. Just return to it when you're ready – your path is yours to walk, in your time.

Your Pride Statement

I've completed my 12 actions from *The Complete Anti-Inflammatory Guide*. I took action. I stayed curious. I made time.

I'm proud of what I've started - and I'm not stopping here.

(Sign here if you'd like a reminder that you did this):

Signature: _____ Date: _____

Join the Community & Celebrate Your Progress. Want to mark your progress in a tangible way?

Once you've completed your 12 actions, visit our website to fill in a short form and receive your personalised **Master of Self-Care Certificate**. You'll be joining a growing community of like-minded readers who are choosing to take consistent, intentional steps toward better health.

Please Visit: www.selfcarenation.co.uk or scan the QR code below to take your first intentional steps toward better health.

Because small steps deserve recognition — and you've taken twelve.

Chapter One
Understanding Chronic Inflammation

Chronic inflammation is often invisible

One crisp autumn morning, a close friend – a vibrant woman in her fifties – recounted how she had always attributed her constant fatigue and occasional aches to the inevitabilities of aging. She managed a demanding career, a bustling household, and the usual stressors of suburban life. It was only during a routine check-up that her doctor mentioned chronic inflammation after reviewing her symptoms and blood tests. Though she had heard the term before, she had never fully understood its implications.

As we chatted over coffee, she expressed relief in finally having an explanation for her discomfort. Though overwhelming, understanding chronic inflammation initially brought a sense of reassurance and hope. Her story underscores an important reality – chronic inflammation is often invisible, quietly influencing our health in ways we don't immediately recognize.

1.1 The Silent Fire: What is Chronic Inflammation?

Inflammation isn't inherently harmful. Acute inflammation is the body's natural defense mechanism, activated by an injury or infection. It manifests as redness, heat, swelling, and pain, indicating that the immune system is responding. In this process, immune cells rush to the affected area, neutralizing threats and initiating healing. Once the body recovers, acute inflammation subsides, allowing normal function to resume.

Chronic inflammation, however, behaves differently. Instead of resolving, it lingers for months or even years, keeping the immune system in a constant state of low-grade activation. This persistent immune response, a natural defense mechanism, turns against the body over time, damaging tissues and increasing the risk of serious diseases.

At the core of chronic inflammation is the continuous release of cytokines – small messenger proteins that regulate immune responses and call the immune troops. While cytokines play an essential role in the body's healing and defense, their persistent overproduction leads to tissue breakdown rather than repair. In simpler terms, it's like having too many over-zealous soldiers (cytokines) on the battlefield (your body) all the time, causing damage to your own territory(tissues) instead of just fighting off the enemies (infections). This prolonged immune activation, driven by cytokines, has been linked to cardiovascular disease, diabetes, autoimmune disorders, and neurodegenerative conditions.

Many people, like my friend, mistake fatigue, joint pain, and digestive discomfort for normal aging or stress. Because chronic inflammation doesn't cause immediate or noticeable symptoms, it is often dismissed or ignored. However, understanding the signs and symptoms of chronic inflammation can help us detect it early, empowering us to take proactive steps to prevent severe health conditions from developing.

Think of chronic inflammation like a small leak in the roof. At first, it's barely noticeable, just a minor drip. However ,over time, the slow accumulation of damage weakens the structure, leading to costly and sometimes irreversible consequences. The same applies to chronic inflammation. It silently damages tissues, weakens immune defenses, and accelerates aging, much like a leaky roof weakens a building's structure.

Key Consequences of Chronic Inflammation:

- Accelerates cellular aging – Collagen breakdown leads to wrinkles and skin sagging.

- Slows tissue repair – Muscles, joints, and organs recover more slowly.

- Impairs brain function – Contributes to brain fog and cognitive decline.

- Increases risk of common chronic diseases – Linked to conditions such as heart disease, type 2 diabetes, obesity, arthritis, and certain cancers.

The good news is that this process is reversible with proactive lifestyle changes. By making informed choices about diet, exercise, stress management, and sleep, we can take control and reverse the effects of chronic inflammation, empowering ourselves to lead healthier lives.

1.2 Root Causes: Triggers of Chronic Inflammation

Our daily choices often shape our body's inflammatory response without realizing it. Diet, in particular, plays a significant role. Many people rely on ultra-processed, high-sugar foods due to convenience, such as fizzy drinks, sugary cereals, fast food, and packaged snacks. These foods introduce excess simple carbohydrates, unhealthy fats, and artificial additives. Over time, this dietary pattern disrupts blood sugar levels, increases oxidative stress, and triggers inflammation.

Taste preferences often influence food choices, but they can be retrained. The more we expose our taste buds to natural, unprocessed ingredients, the more we shift toward healthier eating habits. This transformation reduces inflammation and improves energy levels, digestion, and well-being.

The Role of Physical Inactivity

While diet plays a crucial role in inflammation, how much we move is another major factor.

Regular physical activity is not just about weight control; it is critical in regulating immune function and reducing inflammation. When we move, our body releases myokines – anti-inflammatory molecules that help counteract the effects of chronic inflammation.

In contrast, prolonged inactivity leads to visceral fat accumulation, which secretes inflammatory cytokines and pushes the body into a chronic inflammatory state. In simpler terms, it's like having a fat factory (visceral fat) in your body that produces soldiers (inflammatory cytokines) all the time, causing inflammation throughout your body.

Many office workers who spend hours sitting report fatigue, joint stiffness, and muscle aches. The lack of movement restricts blood flow and nutrient delivery to tissues, worsening inflammation. Over time, this cycle of inactivity and inflammation can lead to metabolic disorders and reduced mobility.

Wider Determinants of Health

Beyond diet and activity, environmental and genetic factors contribute to inflammation. Air pollution, water contaminants, and household chemicals introduce toxins that infiltrate the body and trigger immune responses. People living in urban, high-pollution areas often experience higher rates of inflammation-related illnesses such as asthma, cardiovascular disease, and autoimmune disorders.

Genetics also plays a role. Some individuals are predisposed to stronger inflammatory responses due to inherited markers. However, emerging research in epigenetics, studying how our environment and lifestyle can influence gene expression, suggests that lifestyle modifications – such as diet, exercise, stress management, and sleep – can alter gene expression and reduce inflammation. While genetics may set the foundation, proactive choices can override many inherited risks.

The Impact of Stress & Mental Health

Stress is another major trigger. Chronic stress leads to elevated cortisol levels, which fuel inflammation over time. Anxiety and depression are also associated with higher levels of inflammatory markers. The mind and body are deeply connected – emotional distress, linked to stress hormone, cortisol, can manifest physically as inflammation.

Mindfulness practices, relaxation techniques, and social support can significantly reduce inflammation and improve mental and physical health.

Medications & Inflammation

While medications are often necessary, some can contribute to inflammation if misused. Nonsteroidal anti-inflammatory drugs (NSAIDs), commonly used for pain relief, may disrupt gut health when taken frequently. These drugs can erode the intestinal lining, triggering low-grade gut inflammation.

Antibiotic overuse is another concern. While antibiotics are essential for fighting bacterial infections, they can disturb the gut microbiome, allowing harmful bacteria to thrive and promote inflammation. This highlights the importance of balanced medication use and gut-friendly practices like probiotics and fiber-rich diets.

The Cellular Cost of Inflammation

Here's something we don't often think about: every cell in your body has a life cycle. It's born, it does its job, and eventually it's replaced. But the quality of each new cell depends entirely on the internal environment it's created in.

If your body is inflamed, stressed, or poorly nourished, new cells are formed under pressure. They're more likely to be weak, dysfunctional, or inflamed from the start. But when your internal environment is calm and supported - with good nutrition, rest, and movement - your body produces stronger, healthier cells. That's the foundation of lasting vitality.

Obesity adds to this challenge. Visceral fat isn't just excess weight - it's biologically active tissue that pumps out inflammatory chemicals. These drive chronic, low-grade inflammation that damages tissues, disrupts hormones, and weakens the quality of new cells. It becomes a self-perpetuating cycle: inflammation leads to poor cell health, which leads to more dysfunction.

That's why improving your internal environment - through lifestyle, not just calorie counting – matters. You're not just losing weight or reducing symptoms. *You're upgrading the next generation of cells your body produces, one day at a time.*

1.2A Fitness Is Not Enough: Why Immunological Strength Matters

Most people believe that physical fitness is the ultimate marker of health. A lean body, strong muscles, and endurance are celebrated everywhere – from magazine covers to gym ads. But the truth is more profound and more urgent: Fitness is not enough. Without a strong and balanced immune system, even the fittest bodies can falter.

When I was recovering from COVID-19, two news headlines appeared within days of each other. One told the uplifting story of a 70-year-old patient, frail but resilient, walking out of the hospital after surviving the virus. The other was heartbreaking: a 40-year-old marathon runner, celebrated for his stamina and health, lost his life after contracting COVID-19.

How could this happen? How could someone younger, stronger, and seemingly in peak physical shape not survive, while an older person could?

The answer lies in immunological fitness – the strength, flexibility, and resilience of the immune system.

Physical fitness and immunological fitness are related but distinct.

You can have incredible cardiovascular endurance yet have an immune system that's overburdened, inflamed, or poorly regulated.

On the other hand, someone with modest physical capacity but a well-nourished, balanced immune system can withstand severe infections, heal faster, and recover more fully.

True health means nurturing both:

- The body's ability to move and perform, and

- The body's ability to defend, repair, and regenerate.

Immunological fitness is built not just through exercise, but through everything we discuss in this guide:

Nutrition, sleep, stress management, gut health, inflammation control, and emotional well-being.

It is the foundation that determines whether your body responds with resilience – or breaks under pressure.

The tragedy of COVID-19 taught us a powerful lesson:

- Muscles alone can't protect you.

- Running marathons alone can't protect you.

- Strength and stamina are important, but they must be accompanied by an immune system that is ready, adaptive, and calm.

Mental Fitness: The Hidden Pillar of Immunity

Physical fitness strengthens your body, but mental fitness protects your immune system from the inside out. Chronic stress, worry, and emotional burnout weaken your body's natural defenses, leaving you more vulnerable to infections and slower recovery.

Building mental resilience – through mindfulness, gratitude, meaningful connection, and stress management – is not a luxury. It is a crucial pillar of true immunity.

Your immune system listens to your mind as much as your muscles. Nourish both, and you build a fortress from within.

In the chapters ahead, we will keep this broader definition of health in mind. Because achieving vitality isn't just about pushing your entire body harder – it's about healing it, feeding it, and supporting it from the inside out.

1.3 Health Implications: Chronic Diseases Linked to Inflammation

Chronic inflammation does more than cause discomfort – it lays the foundation for some of the most prevalent and debilitating diseases. From heart disease to metabolic disorders, autoimmune conditions, and neurological decline, inflammation acts as a common denominator, exacerbating health risks and accelerating disease progression.

The Role of Inflammation in Major Diseases

• Cardiovascular Disease – Inflammation is a critical driver of atherosclerosis, the process by which plaque accumulates in the arteries. It begins when inflammatory cells and lipids embed themselves in artery walls, causing them to thicken and harden. Over time, these plaques can rupture, leading to blood clots that block circulation, triggering heart attacks or strokes. Inflammation fuels this process by continuously activating the immune system, worsening arterial damage, and increasing the risk of life-threatening events.

- Type 2 Diabetes & Insulin Resistance – The link between chronic inflammation and type 2 diabetes is profound. Inflammatory cytokines interfere with insulin signaling, preventing cells from properly absorbing glucose. As insulin resistance develops, the body struggles to regulate blood sugar levels, leading to persistent hyperglycemia (high blood sugar). This cycle of inflammation and metabolic dysfunction increases the risk of nerve damage, kidney disease, and cardiovascular complications. Addressing inflammation through dietary and lifestyle changes is crucial in preventing and managing diabetes.

- Autoimmune Disorders – Conditions like rheumatoid arthritis, lupus, and multiple sclerosis arise when the immune system mistakenly attacks the body's tissues. Inflammation plays a dual role here – it is both a symptom and a driving force behind these conditions. Cytokines fuel this misdirected immune response, leading to joint destruction, organ damage, and systemic symptoms like fatigue and brain fog. Understanding these diseases as manifestations of dysregulated inflammation allows for better management through targeted therapies, stress reduction, and lifestyle interventions.

- Metabolic Syndrome & Obesity – Excess weight – especially visceral fat stored around the abdomen – contributes to chronic inflammation. Fat cells aren't just passive storage units; they secrete pro-inflammatory cytokines, promoting a cycle of metabolic dysfunction. This inflammatory burden increases the risk of high blood pressure, insulin resistance, abnormal cholesterol levels, and the hallmark symptoms of metabolic syndrome. Chronic inflammation makes weight loss harder and disrupts hormones that regulate hunger and metabolism, further complicating efforts to achieve a healthy weight.

- Neurological Disorders & Mental Health – Inflammation's impact on the brain is often overlooked, yet it plays a significant role in neurodegenerative diseases and mental health conditions. Research has linked chronic inflammation to Alzheimer's disease, where inflammatory molecules contribute to amyloid plaque build up, impairing neural communication and accelerating cognitive decline.

Additionally, inflammation is associated with depression and anxiety. Studies show that individuals with these conditions often have elevated inflammatory markers, including C-reactive protein (CRP) and interleukin-6 (IL-6). This suggests that chronic inflammation may influence mood disorders by disrupting neurotransmitter function and increasing oxidative stress in the brain.

The Role of Nutrition in Disease Prevention

A study by Massachusetts General Hospital, in collaboration with Community Servings, revealed that providing medically tailored meals to high-risk Medicaid and Medicare patients significantly reduced hospitalizations and healthcare costs. Patients receiving anti-inflammatory meals had a 16% reduction in overall medical expenses, highlighting the diet's decisive role in preventing and managing disease.

By addressing inflammation through targeted lifestyle interventions, individuals can lower disease risk, improve quality of life, and enhance longevity.

1.4 Detecting the Invisible: Symptoms & Early Detection

Inflammation often develops quietly, masked by symptoms easily overlooked or misattributed to stress, aging, or lifestyle factors. Because chronic inflammation does not always cause acute pain or visible distress, it can persist for years before being diagnosed.

Common Warning Signs of Chronic Inflammation

• Persistent Fatigue – Tiredness that lingers despite rest and proper sleep.

• Digestive Issues – Bloating, irregular bowel movements, or symptoms resembling Irritable Bowel Syndrome(IBS).

• Brain Fog – Difficulty concentrating, forgetfulness, and mental exhaustion.

• Joint Pain & Muscle Stiffness – Persistent aches that worsen over time.

• Frequent Infections – Increased susceptibility to colds, flu, and other illnesses.

Because these symptoms can be vague or fluctuate, many people fail to connect them to chronic inflammation.

Medical Tests for Detecting Chronic Inflammation

To identify inflammation, healthcare providers use specific diagnostic tests:

• C-Reactive Protein (CRP) Test – This simple blood test measures systemic inflammation levels. Elevated CRP suggests ongoing inflammation and increased disease risk.

• Erythrocyte Sedimentation Rate (ESR) – This measures how quickly red blood cells settle in a test tube, indicating inflammation in the body.

• Interleukin-6 (IL-6) Levels – Higher IL-6 levels are associated with diabetes, heart disease, and cognitive decline.

While these tests provide valuable insights, they are not standalone diagnostic tools. Instead, they help build a broader picture of inflammatory health, guiding doctors in identifying underlying causes and recommending appropriate interventions. Ask your GP about CRP and ESR tests if you suspect chronic inflammation.

The Role of Self-Assessment

Beyond medical testing, self-awareness plays a crucial role in early detection.

- Keeping a Health Journal – Tracking diet, activity levels, and symptoms can help identify triggers that contribute to inflammation.
- Monitoring Energy & Mood – Noting fatigue, concentration, and motivation fluctuations can offer insights into inflammatory patterns.
- Evaluating Diet & Lifestyle Choices – Identifying which foods, stressors, or habits worsen symptoms can guide healthier adjustments.

By tuning in to these early warning signals, individuals can take preventive action before chronic inflammation leads to serious health complications.

The Importance of Professional Guidance

A multidisciplinary approach is essential in tackling chronic inflammation, with each healthcare professional playing a distinct yet complementary role:

- Doctors – Diagnose and oversee treatment plans, ensuring that medical interventions address symptoms and root causes.
- Pharmacists – As highly trained clinicians accessible on the high street, pharmacists provide expert advice on drug interactions, medication-induced nutrient deficiencies, and lifestyle modifications that enhance treatment outcomes.
- Dietitians & Nutritionists – Develop tailored dietary strategies, focusing on anti-inflammatory foods that support long-term health and disease prevention.
- Physiotherapists – Guide patients in movement-based interventions to reduce inflammation, improve mobility, and enhance overall physical function.

This collaborative model ensures that patients receive well-rounded, proactive care that integrates medical treatment and preventive strategies, empowering them to take control of their health.

1.5 Beyond Diet and Exercise: The Hidden Contributors to Inflammation

When discussing chronic inflammation, the conversation typically revolves around diet, exercise, and stress management. While these factors are essential, they're not the only influence on inflammation. Many subtle aspects of our lives quietly impact our health. Insights from the Institute for Integrative Nutrition's Circle of Life highlight how emotional and social factors significantly affect our body's inflammatory responses.

Joy, Happiness, and Emotional Well-being: The Most Overlooked Anti-Inflammatory Forces

When we talk about health, we often forget the power of joy, laughter, and emotional safety - but these are potent anti-inflammatory forces. Happiness does more than lift our spirits – it actively boosts our immune health. Positive emotions like joy, gratitude, and satisfaction directly reduce cortisol levels, a hormone closely associated with inflammation. Activities that spark joy, such as laughter, dancing, gardening, or painting, have been scientifically linked to lower inflammation markers.

For instance, a study in Psychosomatic Medicine discovered that participants engaging in joyful hobbies regularly experienced notably lower inflammatory responses. By intentionally including joyful moments in our daily routines - listening to favorite music, walking in nature, or pursuing creative interests - we create a powerful shield against chronic inflammation.

Social Connections and Relationships

Human beings are social by nature, and the quality of our relationships profoundly influences our health. Firm, supportive connections enhance our resilience, making coping with life's ups and downs easier. On the other hand, loneliness and social isolation quietly fuel inflammation. Studies have shown that individuals experiencing loneliness exhibit higher inflammation markers like IL-6 and C-reactive protein (CRP).

Engaging regularly with family, friends, or community groups activates brain pathways that reduce stress and inflammation. Simple actions – such as joining local clubs, volunteering, or making regular calls to friends – can profoundly improve emotional and physical health.

Spirituality and Sense of Purpose

Spirituality and a sense of purpose are more than abstract ideas – they tangibly impact our physical health. Individuals who consistently engage in spiritual practices or have a strong sense of purpose report lower inflammation levels. Living with purpose promotes emotional stability, helps manage stress, and reduces chronic inflammation.

Research published in Brain, Behavior, and Immunity found that regular mindfulness and meditation significantly lowered inflammation markers like TNF-alpha and CRP. Practicing mindfulness meditation, prayer, or even community volunteering can greatly enhance emotional well-being and reduce inflammation.

Creativity and Play

Play and creativity aren't just for children - they're critical to adult health, too. Activities such as painting, writing, dancing, or playing games stimulate relaxation centers in the brain, reducing stress hormones and inflammatory cytokines.

Studies on art therapy have consistently found that participants experience reduced stress and lower inflammation levels. Integrating brief creative moments into our daily schedules - journaling, sketching, playing music, or exploring new hobbies - can significantly reduce chronic inflammation. Creativity offers an accessible and enjoyable path to better health.

Home Environment

Our everyday living spaces directly, yet often overlooked, affect inflammation. A home environment characterized by clutter, chaos, or emotional tension subtly but persistently elevates stress levels, contributing to chronic inflammation. Conversely, creating a calm, organized, and peaceful home reduces stress hormones, helping our immune systems stay balanced.

Research published in Personality and Social Psychology Bulletin showed that individuals who described their homes as cluttered or stressful had elevated cortisol levels. Simple practices like decluttering spaces, adding plants, increasing natural lighting, or setting aside quiet areas for relaxation can transform our homes into sanctuaries that actively reduce inflammation.

Career Satisfaction and Financial Security

Work-related stress and financial anxiety are potent drivers of inflammation, yet their impact is frequently overlooked. Chronic dissatisfaction with a job or persistent financial stress raises stress hormone levels, creating ongoing inflammation.

Research in Occupational and Environmental Medicine highlights how chronic job dissatisfaction elevates inflammation markers. Similarly, ongoing financial anxiety significantly increases inflammatory cytokines such as IL-6. Taking proactive steps to improve career satisfaction, such as developing new skills, achieving better work-life balance, or seeking financial counseling, can notably reduce these inflammatory stresses and improve overall health.

Practical Steps to Holistic Health

Recognizing the vast array of factors contributing to inflammation empowers us to take holistic action. Effective inflammation management means nurturing social bonds, embracing joyful activities, cultivating a sense of purpose, engaging creatively, creating supportive home environments, and pursuing career and financial well-being. Each aspect interconnects, forming a protective network that helps prevent and reverse chronic inflammation.

Conclusion

By broadening our focus beyond diet and exercise, we discover new pathways to sustained health and effectively manage chronic inflammation through a comprehensive, integrative approach. By understanding and addressing these hidden influences, we prepare ourselves to confront another critical aspect of inflammation – medication-related nutrient deficiencies – explored in depth in the next chapter: "The Hidden Pandemic."

Your Healing Reflection:

- Which symptoms or health issues might be linked to chronic inflammation?
- How do they affect your day-to-day well-being?

Please complete the 'I will ...' statement on page 5.

CHAPTER TWO

THE HIDDEN PANDEMIC – HOW MEDICATIONS ARE FUELING NUTRIENT DEFICIENCIES AND INFLAMMATION

The Unseen Consequences of Long-Term Medication Use

In the A&E department, a man in his sixties clutches his chest, confused and exhausted. He is on six different medications – each prescribed to manage a different condition – yet he keeps getting sicker. How did he get here? For decades, we've been told that medications are the answer to our health problems. Yet many people take them for years – sometimes decades – without realizing that their persistent fatigue, joint pain, or cognitive fog might not be signs of ageing or bad luck, but the result of the hidden pandemic. Could it be that the very treatments meant to improve health are also contributing to its decline?

2.1 – The Silent Threat of Drug-Induced Nutrient Deficiency (DIND)

When we think of medication side effects, we often picture nausea, headaches, or dizziness – the common adverse effects listed in patient information leaflets. However, some of the most serious long-term consequences of medications are never mentioned. One of these is Drug-Induced Nutrient Deficiency (DIND), a condition that develops slowly and silently, eroding health over months or years.

Many people who take long-term medications experience fatigue, brain fog, or muscle weakness, but these symptoms are often dismissed as aging, stress, or the progression of the disease itself. In reality, they may be warning signs of nutrient depletion caused by prescription drugs.

'To Err Is Human' – Unrecognized Medication Risks and the Need for Awareness

More than two decades ago, the landmark 1999 Institute of Medicine (IOM) report, To Err Is Human, exposed a shocking reality: medical errors were responsible for tens of thousands of preventable deaths annually in U.S. hospitals. The report led to sweeping changes in patient safety, hospital protocols, and medication management. However, it failed to address a more insidious and long-term risk – the hidden impact of medications depleting vital nutrients, increasing the risk of chronic disease, and silently worsening health over time.

DIND is an iatrogenic disease – one caused by medical treatment itself. Yet, unlike medication overdoses or drug interactions, it remains unmonitored mainly and under-diagnosed.

Armed with knowledge about the risks, patients can advocate for their health and demand better monitoring and management of their medications. This underlines the urgent need for healthcare reform to address this hidden crisis and ensure better patient outcomes.

Pharmacists are not required to flag potential DIND risks during dispensing. This lack of awareness means that millions of people suffer from unexplained symptoms, unaware that their medications may be to blame. However, with increased knowledge and vigilance, these drug-induced nutrient deficiencies are preventable, empowering patients and healthcare professionals alike.

2.2 – The Growing Burden of Preventable Diseases & Medication Overload

The Escalating Health Crisis of Chronic Disease & Polypharmacy

The global burden of chronic diseases – such as hypertension, diabetes, cardiovascular diseases, and arthritis – has surged in the past few decades. Once considered diseases of old age, these conditions appear earlier in life due to poor diet, sedentary lifestyles, and environmental stressors. The response? Widespread prescribing of medications, often for long-term or lifelong use.

In the U.S., 45% of adults are living with at least one chronic disease, and many are prescribed multiple medications.

In the UK, over half of adults aged 65+ take five or more medications daily (polypharmacy).

But here's the problem: many of these medications, while effective at managing symptoms, actively deplete essential nutrients, worsening long-term health outcomes. For instance, certain diuretics can deplete potassium and magnesium, while some acid-reducing medications can reduce vitamin B12 absorption.

We are not just medicating chronic disease – we are silently creating new health challenges by depleting the very nutrients the body needs to function optimally.

The Hidden Cost of Medication-Driven Nutrient Loss

When patients start experiencing new symptoms—fatigue, depression, muscle weakness, or brain fog – after years on medication, they are rarely checked for nutrient depletion. Instead, they are often prescribed additional medications to manage their new symptoms. This cycle, called the Prescription Cascade, leads to:

- Higher risk of drug interactions and side effects.
- Increased reliance on medications rather than addressing underlying deficiencies.
- Rising healthcare costs due to preventable complications.

Case Example: A Common Polypharmacy Scenario

A patient with high blood pressure is prescribed a diuretic to manage their condition. Over time, the diuretic depletes potassium and magnesium, leading to muscle cramps and fatigue. Instead of addressing this deficiency, they are prescribed a muscle relaxant and antidepressant, further depleting B vitamins and CoQ10. The patient, unaware of the impact of nutrient loss, feels worse and is now on three medications instead of one.

Post-COVID Mental Health Crisis & Medication Dependence

The COVID-19 pandemic has led to a sharp rise in mental health disorders, with millions turning to antidepressants, benzodiazepines, and antipsychotics for relief. However, these medications also contribute to DIND by depleting:

- B vitamins – essential for brain function, nerve health, and mood regulation.
- Magnesium – a critical mineral for reducing anxiety and muscle relaxation.
- CoenzymeQ10 (CoQ10) – supports cellular energy and protects against fatigue.

Antidepressant use has increased by 20% globally since the pandemic. Yet, nutrient depletion in psychiatric patients remains an overlooked issue.

How many people are being misdiagnosed with worsening depression when, in reality, they are experiencing medication-induced nutrient depletion?

2.3 – The Economic Costs of DIND & The Healthcare System's Blind Spot

The Rising Financial Burden of Chronic Disease & Medication Dependency

The economic impact of chronic disease and medication dependency is staggering. Governments and healthcare systems worldwide spend billions annually managing conditions that, in many cases, could be prevented or improved through better nutritional awareness. However, the hidden costs of drug-induced nutrient deficiency (DIND) remain ignored mainly in financial assessments of healthcare sustainability.

In the UK, the NHS spends an estimated £14.7 billion annually on treating patients harmed by medication errors and adverse drug effects – but this figure does not account for nutrient depletion-related health decline, which often leads to additional medical treatments.

The U.S. spends over $500 billion annually on chronic disease management, with a significant portion linked to medication side effects – yet DIND is rarely monitored or factored into treatment costs.

The Unseen Costs of DIND on Patient Health & Quality of Life

The consequences of long-term medication use without proper nutrient monitoring go beyond financial strain. Patients unknowingly suffer the effects of nutrient depletion, leading to:

- Increased doctor visits due to unexplained fatigue, depression, or muscle pain.

- More hospitalizations from medication-induced heart problems, osteoporosis, or nerve damage.
- Workforce productivity loss as employees experience cognitive decline and chronic fatigue.
- Higher disability claims due to conditions worsened by silent nutrient deficiencies.

We're not just managing chronic disease with medications – we're creating a silent epidemic of nutrient depletion that is worsening public health outcomes.

The Healthcare System's Blind Spot: Why DIND is Not Monitored

- No routine screenings: Most healthcare providers do not routinely test for medication-induced nutrient deficiencies. Blood tests for key nutrients such as magnesium, B12, vitamin D, and CoQ10 are rarely included in standard care.
- Lack of awareness in prescribing: Doctors focus on managing symptoms of chronic disease but are rarely trained to consider nutrient depletion as a contributing factor.
- Pharmacists are not required to intervene: While pharmacists play a key role in dispensing medications, they are not mandated to counsel patients on potential nutrient depletion.

The result? Millions of patients suffer avoidable health complications that could be prevented with simple dietary and supplement interventions.

2.4 – Dysbiosis, Gut-Brain Axis, and DIND's Role in Inflammation

The Gut-Brain Axis: How Medication Disrupts Mood & Cognition

The gut and brain are deeply connected – a relationship known as the gut-brain axis. This two-way communication system regulates mood, cognition, and overall mental well-being. Yet, many medications disrupt gut health, indirectly impacting mental resilience and cognitive function.

Proton pump inhibitors (PPIs), antibiotics, and antidepressants alter the gut microbiome, reducing beneficial bacteria needed for neurotransmitter production.

When the microbiome is compromised, serotonin and dopamine synthesis is affected, worsening symptoms of anxiety and depression.

Medications that damage gut health and impact brain function:

- PPIs & Antacids – Reduce stomach acid, impairing nutrient absorption (B12, magnesium, iron).
- Antibiotics – Kill beneficial gut bacteria, reducing serotonin production.
- SSRIs & Antipsychotics – Alter microbial diversity, affecting the gut's ability to regulate inflammation.

Medication-induced gut imbalances and nutrient depletion may worsen many psychiatric symptoms linked to depression or anxiety.

Medication-Induced Dysbiosis & Inflammation

When gut bacteria become imbalanced (dysbiosis), inflammation spreads throughout the body – including the brain. Chronic inflammation, fuelled by nutrient deficiencies, is a hidden driver of mental health disorders, autoimmune diseases, and metabolic dysfunction.

- Dysbiosis leads to a leaky gut, allowing inflammatory compounds to enter the bloodstream and trigger systemic inflammation.
- Inflammation disrupts brain function, contributing to brain fog, cognitive decline, and fatigue.
- Chronic medication use without microbiome support increases long-term disease risk.

Inflammation doesn't just cause pain – it impairs brain function, metabolic health, and emotional well-being.

Supporting Gut Health to Reduce DIND's Impact

To counteract medication-induced dysbiosis, patients should:

- Consume more fermented foods (kimchi, sauerkraut, yogurt) to support gut diversity.
- Include prebiotic-rich foods (garlic, onions, bananas) to feed beneficial bacteria.
- Avoid excessive processed foods & sugars, which fuel harmful gut bacteria.
- Consider probiotic supplements if on long-term antibiotics, PPIs, or antidepressants.

Protecting gut health is crucial for preventing the long-term inflammatory effects of DIND.

What we eat directly impacts inflammation, and inflammation is at the root of many chronic diseases - conditions that, in many cases, can be prevented, improved, or even put into remission with lifestyle changes. But here's the catch: when these diseases are managed solely with long-term medications, the drugs meant to help can strip the body of essential nutrients, fuelling more inflammation and opening the door to new health problems. This creates a cycle where medications lead to nutrient loss, which leads to more illness, more prescriptions, and, ultimately, iatrogenic disease – health complications caused by the treatment itself. Breaking this cycle starts with awareness and addressing the impact of medications on our nutrition and overall well-being.

2.5 – Ethical Implications, 'First, Do No Harm,' and Patient-Centered Care

The Ethical Obligation: First, Do No Harm

The fundamental principle of medical ethics - "First, do no harm" (Primum non nocere)—requires healthcare providers to prioritize patient safety above all else. However, drug-induced nutrient deficiency (DIND) represents an apparent failure in this duty.

Medications meant to heal can simultaneously harm the body by creating nutrient imbalances, fuelling inflammation, and triggering secondary health problems. Yet, these effects are rarely disclosed, screened for, or addressed in standard medical practice.

Why DIND is a Patient Safety Issue:

☐ It is preventable – Nutrient depletion is not an inevitable consequence of medication use; it can be identified and corrected.

☐ It is overlooked – Routine medical care does not monitor for DIND, leaving patients vulnerable.

☐ It contributes to new diseases – Many patients develop secondary health conditions that could have been avoided.

"If a prescribed drug depletes essential nutrients that sustain life, is it truly helping the patient - or creating a new, hidden form of harm?"

The Patient's Right to Informed Consent

Patients have the right to know about all potential risks associated with their medications - including nutrient depletion and its consequences.

But currently, DIND is not listed in standard drug safety warnings, nor is it commonly discussed in consultations.

What Needs to Change?

☐ Doctors must disclose potential nutrient depletion risks when prescribing long-term medication.

☐ Pharmacists should provide guidance on nutrient monitoring, dietary support, and supplementation.

☐ Healthcare policies should integrate nutrient screening into chronic disease management protocols.

Patients should never have to suffer preventable harm due to lack of information. Empowering individuals with knowledge is the first step in preventing DIND.

Shifting to a Patient-Centered Model of Care

Traditional healthcare focuses on treating symptoms, not addressing root causes. A patient-centered approach would:

☐ Prioritize prevention over reaction – Identifying nutrient depletion early would prevent long-term health consequences.

☐ Encourage collaboration – Physicians, pharmacists, and dietitians must work together to monitor patient well-being.

☐ Educate patients – Clear, accessible information on DIND should be included in medication consultations and online resources.

A proactive, rather than reactive, healthcare model can prevent harm, improve outcomes, and reduce unnecessary medication use.

2.6 – Actionable Strategies for Preventing & Managing DIND

While DIND is a hidden but serious health issue, it is not inevitable. By taking proactive steps, patients and healthcare professionals can work together to minimize the risks and improve health outcomes.

Healthcare Providers: The Role of Doctors, Pharmacists & Dietitians

Healthcare professionals must take the lead in integrating DIND screening into routine care. This means:

☐ Doctors should evaluate nutrient depletion risks before prescribing long-term medication.

☐ Pharmacists should counsel patients on how to counteract nutrient loss.

☐ Dietitians should develop personalized nutrition plans to support patients on multiple medications.

Key Strategies for Healthcare Providers:

☐ Incorporate routine nutrient screening – Test for B12, magnesium, vitamin D, CoQ10, and other essential nutrients in patients on long-term medications.

- Use a risk-based approach – Identify which patients are at highest risk (e.g., those on PPIs, statins, antidepressants, and diuretics).
- Educate patients about drug-nutrient interactions – Provide easy-to-understand guides on how medications affect nutrient absorption.

A patient should never suffer from preventable health complications from unmonitored nutrient depletion.

Patients: How to Take an Active Role in Preventing DIND

Patients must become advocates for their health. This means:
- Asking the right questions before starting a new medication.
- Tracking symptoms to detect early warning signs of nutrient depletion.
- Requesting routine nutrient testing from their doctor.

What Every Patient Should Ask Their Doctor or Pharmacist:
- "Does this medication deplete any essential nutrients?"
- "Should I take any dietary supplements or make dietary changes?"
- "What symptoms should I watch for that might indicate nutrient loss?"
- "Can I have regular blood tests to monitor for deficiencies?"

Patient empowerment starts with knowledge. The more informed individuals are, the better they can protect their health.

The Role of Diet & Supplementation in Combating DIND

Diet is one of the most potent tools in mitigating the effects of medication-induced nutrient depletion.
- Anti-inflammatory foods help counteract oxidative stress and support cellular health.
- Nutrient-dense whole foods can replenish lost vitamins and minerals.
- Targeted supplementation can restore balance when diet alone is insufficient.

Best Dietary Approaches for Patients on Long-Term Medications:
- For Magnesium Depletion – Eat dark leafy greens, nuts, seeds, and avocados.
- For B12 Deficiency – Include grass-fed meats, eggs, dairy, or B12 supplements.
- For CoQ10 Loss – Consume cold-water fish, organ meats (liver, kidneys etc), and CoQ10 supplements.
- For Iron & Folate Depletion – Eat lentils, spinach, red meat, and fortified cereals.
- For Gut Health Support – Include fermented foods like yogurt, kefir, kimchi, and probiotics.

A well-structured diet can significantly reduce the risks associated with medication use.

2.7 – Final Thoughts & Call to Action for Healthcare Reform

The Urgent Need for Change in How We Manage Medication Side Effects

Drug-Induced Nutrient Deficiency (DIND) is an unspoken crisis in modern medicine. Millions of people worldwide suffer unexplained fatigue, cognitive decline, muscle pain, and mental health issues – without realizing their medications are silently depleting essential nutrients.

While medical advancements have extended lives, they have also increased reliance on long-term medication use. The unintended consequence? A silent pandemic of nutrient depletion, fuelling inflammation, preventable diseases, and worsening patient outcomes.

Key Lessons from This Chapter:

- DIND is a widespread but largely unrecognized issue in chronic disease management.
- Medications meant to help can deplete critical nutrients, leading to new health problems.
- The gut-brain axis plays a crucial role in drug interactions and inflammation.
- Doctors, pharmacists, and dietitians must work together to prevent long-term medication damage.
- Patients must become their advocates - asking questions, tracking symptoms, and demanding better care.

Addressing DIND must become a standard part of patient care – not an afterthought.

A Call to Action: How Healthcare Must Change

- Mandatory Nutrient Screening in Long-Term Medication Use - Patients on high-risk drugs should receive regular blood tests for essential vitamins and minerals.
- Integrating Nutritional Therapy into Prescription Protocols - Healthcare providers should recommend dietary changes and supplementation as part of routine care.
- Raising Public Awareness – Governments, medical institutions, and advocacy groups must educate the public on the risks of medication-driven nutrient loss.
- Interdisciplinary Collaboration - Physicians, pharmacists, and dietitians should collaborate to monitor and mitigate the effects of DIND.

If we are genuinely committed to 'First, do no harm,' then recognizing and addressing DIND is not optional - it is an ethical responsibility.

What Patients Can Do Today to Protect Themselves

- Ask questions – Ensure your doctor or pharmacist informs you about nutrient depletion risks before starting a medication.
- Track symptoms - Keep a journal of energy levels, mood, and cognitive function to spot early warning signs of deficiencies.
- Request routine nutrient testing - Advocate for blood tests to check B12, magnesium, CoQ10, vitamin D, and iron levels.
- Adjust your diet accordingly - Prioritize whole foods, gut-friendly nutrition, and anti-inflammatory meals.
- Consider supplementation - If necessary, take targeted supplements to restore balance under medical guidance.

The fight against DIND starts with awareness, action, and accountability.

What we eat directly impacts inflammation, which is at the root of many chronic diseases – conditions that, in many cases, can be prevented, improved, or even put into remission with lifestyle changes. But here's the catch: when these diseases are managed solely with long-term medications, the drugs meant to help can strip the body of essential nutrients, fuelling more inflammation and opening the door to new health problems.

This creates a cycle where medications lead to nutrient loss, which leads to more illness, more medications, and, ultimately, iatrogenic disease – health complications caused by the treatment itself.

Breaking this cycle starts with awareness and addressing the impact of medications on our nutrition and overall well-being.

In the next chapter, we'll explore nutrition's role in healing, diving into food as medicine. We'll uncover how specific dietary choices can reduce inflammation and enhance vitality.

Your journey toward optimal health continues – one step, stretch, and breath at a time.

Your Healing Reflection:

- Can you identify 2–3 habits or exposures in your routine that may be quietly fuelling inflammation?
- What might be the first step in reducing them?

Please complete the 'I will ...' statement on page 5.

Chapter Three

Food is Medicine

Exploring the Healing Power of Nutrition

Picture the comforting scent of a freshly prepared meal filling your kitchen – a symphony of spices and herbs dancing in the air. For many, the kitchen is not just a place for sustenance but a sanctuary for healing. As you navigate the complexities of modern life, juggling work, family, and well-being, the concept of Food is Medicine can revolutionise your health journey. Your decisions at the dining table wield the power to combat inflammation, restore equilibrium, and boost vitality. You are the architect of your health, one meal at a time.

Take Borja, a passionate chef who recently returned from a journey through India, where he spent time visiting health ashrams known for blending ancient wisdom with nutritional science. What he discovered was a revelation: food was not simply a cultural expression or indulgence – it was therapy. At these ashrams, meals were thoughtfully prepared to support digestion, reduce inflammation, and promote overall balance in mind and body. The ingredients – turmeric, ginger, fenugreek, holy basil – were not just flavourful; they were chosen for their healing properties.

Returning home, Borja transformed his kitchen into a wellness lab. Inspired by what he had seen, he began crafting menus that embraced these principles – not only for his own health but for those around him. His cooking changed from performance to purpose. His dinners, once accustomed to rich, decadent meals, found themselves energised and lighter, with some even reporting improvements in sleep and digestion. Borja's experience is a powerful reminder that when we view food through the lens of healing, every recipe becomes a remedy.

This chapter explores how nutrient-dense, anti-inflammatory foods can support your body's natural healing processes. Every meal allows you to take control of your health – one bite at a time.

3.1. The Power of an Anti-Inflammatory Diet

A well-balanced diet forms the bedrock for combating chronic inflammation. While shunning pro-inflammatory triggers, the crux lies in incorporating whole foods with sustained energy, vital nutrients, and immune-boosting properties. This dietary shift can transform your health, one meal at a time.

Macronutrients: Balancing the Essentials

A well-structured plate should contain:

- Whole Grains– Quinoa, oats, and brown rice provide fiber and slow-releasing energy, helping to regulate blood sugar levels and reduce inflammation.
- Lean Proteins – Poultry, fish, and legumes supply essential amino acids without the inflammatory fats found in processed or red meats.
- Healthy Fats – Avocados, olive oil, and nuts support cellular health, reduce inflammation, and promote cardiovascular well-being.

The Fiber Connection: Supporting Gut & Immune Health

Fiber plays a dual role in digestive health and inflammation control. It supports gut bacteria, which in turn regulates immune function. Foods rich in fiber – such as beans, lentils, and leafy greens – help stabilize blood sugar, promote digestion, and keep the gut microbiome balanced.

Antioxidants: Protecting Your Cells

Antioxidants neutralize free radicals – unstable molecules that cause cellular damage and fuel inflammation. Vibrant, colorful foods contain high levels of these potent compounds:

- Berries – Rich in anthocyanins, which combat oxidative stress.
- Dark Chocolate – Contains flavonoids that support heart and brain health.
- Artichokes & Leafy Greens – Aid in detoxification and reduce inflammation.

By including a variety of antioxidant-rich foods in your meals, you strengthen your body's defense system, reducing the risk of inflammatory-related conditions.

3.2. Essential Healing Foods

Some foods stand out as true medicinal powerhouses. These ingredients nourish and actively heal by reducing inflammation and supporting long-term health.

Turmeric & Ginger: Potent Anti-Inflammatory Spices

- Turmeric – Contains curcumin, a bioactive compound with anti-inflammatory and antioxidant properties. When paired with black pepper, curcumin absorption increases significantly.
- Ginger – Helps reduce muscle soreness and inflammation, making it ideal for post-workout recovery and joint health.

Try This: Add turmeric to soups, teas, or curries. Incorporate fresh ginger into stir-fries, herbal teas, or smoothies.

Leafy Greens: Nutrient-Dense Superfoods

Dark leafy greens such as spinach, kale, and Swiss chard provide:

- Vitamin K – Supports bone health and inflammation regulation.
- Vitamin C – A powerful antioxidant that boosts immunity.
- Iron & Calcium – Essential for oxygen transport and muscle function.

Try This: Sauté spinach with garlic and olive oil, blend kale into a smoothie or add Swiss chard to stews.

Fermented Foods: The Gut-Inflammation Link

A healthy gut microbiome is critical for controlling inflammation. Beneficial probiotics in fermented foods help regulate digestion, improve immunity, and reduce inflammatory markers.

- Kimchi & Sauerkraut – Rich in beneficial bacteria that support digestion.
- Yogurt & Kefir – Contain probiotics that maintain gut microbiome balance.

Try This: Include a spoonful of sauerkraut in meals or add yogurt to breakfast bowls.

Omega-3 Fatty Acids: Fighting Inflammation at the Source

Omega-3s are essential for brain, heart, and joint health. These healthy fats lower inflammatory markers and support cognitive function.

- Fatty Fish(salmon, mackerel, sardines) – Provide EPA and DHA, critical for heart and brain health.
- Flaxseeds, Walnuts, & Chia Seeds – Plant-based sources of ALA, another powerful anti-inflammatory omega-3.

Try This: Sprinkle flaxseeds over oatmeal, snack on walnuts, or enjoy grilled salmon with lemon.

3.3. Hydration &Inflammation: The Overlooked Factor

Water is crucial in reducing inflammation, yet it is often overlooked. Hydration helps:
- Flush out toxins.
- Maintain joint lubrication.
- Support digestion and circulation.

Try This: Infuse water with lemon, cucumber, or mint for added flavor. Aim for at least eight glasses of water daily.

3.4. Anti-Inflammatory Diet Checklist

To put these principles into practice, use this checklist when planning meals:
- Whole Grains – Include quinoa, oats, and brown rice.
- Lean Proteins – Opt for fish, poultry, and legumes.
- Healthy Fats – Use olive oil, avocados, and nuts.
- Antioxidant-Rich Foods – Eat berries, dark chocolate, and artichokes.
- High-Fiber Foods – Include beans, lentils, and fruits.
- Omega-3 Sources – Consume fatty fish, walnuts, flaxseeds.
- Hydration –Drink eight glasses of water daily.

By following this checklist, you can create meals that nourish, heal, and sustain your long-term well-being.

3.5. Meal Planning Mastery: Creating Weekly Anti-Inflammatory Menus

Incorporating an anti-inflammatory diet into daily life requires practical strategies. It's one thing to understand the science behind healing foods, but another to consistently apply these principles. This is where meal planning mastery becomes essential. Thoughtful planning ensures that each meal supports your well-being and reduces the stress of last-minute unhealthy choices, providing a sense of security and helping you stay on track without stress.

The Power of Batch Cooking & Smart Meal Prep

One of the simplest ways to stay committed to an anti-inflammatory diet is batch cooking – preparing meals in larger quantities to enjoy throughout the week. Imagine spending a relaxing Sunday afternoon roasting vegetables, cooking quinoa, and grilling lean proteins. When mealtime arrives during the week, you have nutritious, ready-to-go ingredients at your fingertips.

Meal Prep Strategy:

- Cook in Batches – Roast vegetables, grill proteins, and prepare grains in advance.
- Use Portioning – Store pre-prepped meals in individual containers to avoid over-eating.
- Freeze Smartly – Make larger batches of soups or stews and freeze portions for busy days.

Why It Works: Having healthy, pre-prepared meals removes decision fatigue and helps you make nourishing choices effortlessly.

Variety: The Key to Balanced Nutrition & Flavor

One common mistake in healthy eating is falling into a rut, eating the same meals repeatedly. Rotating diverse ingredients keeps your meals nutrient-rich, flavorful, and engaging.

Weekly Ingredient Rotation Strategy:

- Week 1: Mediterranean Focus – Olive oil, tomatoes, chickpeas, fresh herbs.
- Week 2: Asian-Inspired – Bok choy, miso, ginger, tofu, shiitake mushrooms.
- Week 3: Latin American Flavors – Black beans, avocado, quinoa, spicy peppers.

Why It Works: Each cuisine introduces new antioxidants, fiber, and essential nutrients while preventing dietary boredom.

Seasonal & Local Eating: Why It Matters

Eating seasonally and locally enhances nutrient intake and reduces environmental impact. Freshly harvested foods have higher vitamin and antioxidant levels, as they spend less time in transit.

Example of Seasonal Choices:

- Summer: Berries, tomatoes, cucumbers, zucchini.
- Autumn: Apples, sweet potatoes, Brussels sprouts.
- Winter: Citrus fruits, cabbage, root vegetables.
- Spring: Asparagus, strawberries, leafy greens.

Why It Works: Seasonal produce tastes better, provides peak nutrients and supports local farmers.

Flexibility & Personalization: Making It Work for You

Meal planning should fit into your life and not feel restrictive. Adapting meals to preferences makes healthy eating sustainable.

Smart Ingredient Swaps:

- Out of spinach? Use kale or Swiss chard.
- No almonds? Try walnuts or pumpkin seeds.
- Short on time? Use pre-chopped vegetables to save effort.

Why It Works: Personalization ensures your diet remains enjoyable and realistic over time.

Balanced Meal Examples for Anti-Inflammatory Eating

Here's what a day of healing meals could look like:

- Breakfast: Oatmeal topped with blueberries, flaxseeds, and a drizzle of honey.
- Lunch: Quinoa salad with grilled chicken, mixed greens, walnuts, and an olive oil dressing.
- Dinner: Baked salmon with roasted Brussels sprouts and turmeric-spiced sweet potatoes.
- Snacks: Almonds, hummus with carrot sticks or a green smoothie.

Why It Works: Balanced meals provide steady energy, fight inflammation, and taste delicious!

3.6. Real-Life Success: Case Studies of Dietary Transformations

Making dietary changes isn't always easy. Real people have experienced life-changing benefits by adopting an anti-inflammatory lifestyle. Let's explore two stories of transformation and the targeted supplements that helped them achieve even greater results.

Jane's Journey: Overcoming Arthritis Through Food & Supplementation

Jane, a 52-year-old teacher, had had chronic arthritis for over a decade. The stiffness in her joints made everyday activities difficult, and medications offered only temporary relief. Frustrated, she explored natural approaches and discovered the power of an anti-inflammatory diet.

Key Changes Jane Made:
- Eliminated ultra-processed foods – Removed processed sugars, refined grains, and additives.
- Incorporated healing foods – Focused on leafy greens, turmeric, and omega-3-rich fish.
- Monitored triggers – Kept a food diary to identify inflammation-aggravating foods.

Targeted Supplements for Arthritis Relief:
- Turmeric with Black Pepper (Curcumin) – Helped reduce joint inflammation and stiffness.
- Omega-3 Fish Oil – Provided additional anti-inflammatory support for joint health.
- Collagen Peptides – Supported cartilage and connective tissue regeneration.
- Vitamin D & Magnesium – Improved calcium absorption and supported bone strength.

The Results: Within eight weeks, Jane reported less joint pain, improved flexibility, and increased energy. Her diet and supplementation worked together, allowing her to reduce pain medication and regain mobility.

Mark's Story: Reversing Type 2 Diabetes Symptoms with Diet & Supplements

Mark, 48, was diagnosed with type 2 diabetes and struggled with fluctuating blood sugar levels. Seeking a natural way to manage his health, he switched to an anti-inflammatory diet.

Key Changes Mark Made:
- Reduced refined sugars & processed carbs – Focused on whole grains, vegetables, and legumes.
- Balanced macronutrients – Ensured every meal contained fiber, protein, and healthy fats.
- Stayed consistent – Used meal planning and food tracking to stay on course.

Targeted Supplements for Blood Sugar Control:
- Berberine – Helped improve insulin sensitivity and regulate blood sugar.
- Magnesium – Aided in glucose metabolism and reduced inflammation.
- Cinnamon Extract – Assisted in lowering blood sugar spikes after meals.
- Alpha-Lipoic Acid (ALA) – Reduced oxidative stress and supported nerve health.

- Probiotics – Helped balance gut bacteria, which plays a role in blood sugar regulation.

The Results: After six months, Mark's blood sugar stabilized, his energy improved, and his bloating reduced. His doctor noted significant improvements in his metabolic markers, and he was able to reduce his reliance on diabetes medication.

3.7. Why Supplements Matter in an Anti-Inflammatory Approach

While diet remains the foundation of healing, supplements act as powerful reinforcements, particularly in cases of:
- Chronic conditions that require additional support.
- Nutrient deficiencies caused by medications or lifestyle factors.
- Individuals struggling to obtain key nutrients from diet alone.

Important Note: Always consult a healthcare professional before starting new supplements to ensure safety, correct dosages, and effectiveness for your unique needs.

3.8. Overcoming Common Challenges in Dietary Transitions

Switching to an anti-inflammatory diet isn't without hurdles. Many people face barriers – but simple strategies help overcome them.

Jane's Challenge: Adjusting to new flavors.
- Solution: She experimented with herbs and spices to add variety and depth.

Mark's Challenge: Staying consistent with healthy eating while juggling work.
- Solution: He used batch cooking and meal prepping to stay on track.

Lesson: Small, sustainable changes lead to long-term success.

3.9. How to Set Realistic Goals for Sustainable Change

Start Small: Don't overhaul your diet overnight. Instead:
- Week 1: Introduce one new anti-inflammatory food daily.
- Week 2: Reduce processed food intake by 20%.
- Week 3: Plan and prep at least three weekly anti-inflammatory meals.

Track Your Progress: Keep a simple food journal to:
- Identify patterns between food and how you feel.

☐ Stay motivated by tracking improvements in energy, mood, or digestion.

Celebrate Milestones: Acknowledge your progress, whether it's reducing pain, having more energy, or simply feeling better!

3.10 Conclusion: Your Food, Your Medicine

Jane and Mark's experiences demonstrate that small, intentional changes create profound results. The power to heal is in your hands – every meal is an opportunity to reduce inflammation, fuel your body, and reclaim your health.

Borja's story reminds us that healing through food can also be a joyful, creative, and globally inspired process. By learning from traditional healing kitchens and turning his culinary expertise into a wellness mission, he proved that food prepared with intention doesn't just satisfy hunger but restores balance, vitality, and connection.

Next Steps:

Which strategies from this chapter can you apply today?

What small changes can you make this week?

How will you track your progress?

Your health journey starts with a single step – and now, you're on your way to transforming your well-being through food. By combining mindful eating, targeted supplements, and a holistic approach, you can empower your body to heal from within, setting the stage for the next chapter: Movement is Medicine.

Your Healing Reflection:

- Looking at your current eating habits, which foods could you begin reducing, and

- which anti-inflammatory foods would you be excited to explore?

Please complete the 'I will ...' statement on page 5.

Chapter Four

Movement is Medicine

Healing Through the Power of Movement

Imagine this: you've been sitting at your desk for hours, shoulders stiff, neck tense, and lower back aching. It's a sensation many of us know all too well. But what if the solution to this discomfort wasn't a painkiller or a temporary stretch but movement itself – your body's natural way of healing? In an era where sedentary lifestyles have become the norm, movement is more than exercise; it's a transformative force. It can reduce inflammation, physically strengthen the body, and improve overall mental well-being, inspiring you to take charge of your health and wellness journey.

Whether it's a brisk morning walk, a yoga session, or a game of football with friends, every step, stretch, and breath fuels the body's innate ability to heal. In this chapter, we'll explore how movement is an anti-inflammatory powerhouse, examining the wide variety of physical activities available to you, the science behind their healing effects, and ways to incorporate movement into your daily life – no matter how busy your schedule is. This variety empowers you to choose the exercises that best suit your preferences and needs, making your journey to health and wellness personalized and putting you in the driver's seat of your health journey.

4.1. The Science Behind Movement & Inflammation

When you engage in physical activity, your body undergoes a fascinating transformation at the cellular level. Exercise stimulates the release of cytokines, small proteins that regulate immune responses. Among these, IL-6 plays a dual role. While it can act as a pro-inflammatory agent under certain conditions, during exercise, it switches roles and becomes a potent anti-inflammatory molecule. This means that as your muscles contract, they actively help regulate inflammation, reducing levels of harmful inflammatory markers such as TNF-α, which are linked to conditions like arthritis, heart disease, and diabetes.

However, it's important to note that excessive or intense physical activity can lead to overtraining, negatively affecting the body. It's crucial to listen to your body and consult a healthcare professional if you experience persistent pain or discomfort. Additionally, movement triggers the release of endorphins, natural pain-relieving chemicals that improve mood and reduce stress – two key contributors to chronic inflammation. Physical activity also enhances glucose metabolism, helping to stabilize blood sugar levels and reduce the risk of metabolic disorders that fuel inflammation. When you move, you activate a complex network of biological responses that shield your body from chronic inflammation and disease. Moreover, regular physical activity has been shown to reduce symptoms of depression and anxiety and improve overall mental well-being.

4.2 Types of Exercise& Their Anti-Inflammatory Benefits

Not all exercise is created equal, but a well-balanced combination of aerobic activity, strength training, and flexibility exercises provides comprehensive health benefits.

☐ Aerobic Exercise (Cardio): Activities like walking, swimming, cycling, and dancing increase heartrate and circulation, helping to distribute anti-inflammatory agents throughout the body. Regular cardio exercise improves lung function, heart health, and insulin sensitivity, all of which contribute to lowering systemic inflammation.

☐ Resistance Training (Strength Workouts): Weight training and bodyweight exercises – such as squats, lunges, and push-ups – promote muscle growth and metabolic efficiency. Stronger muscles release beneficial cytokines that counteract inflammation and improve overall mobility.

☐ Flexibility & Mobility Work: Stretching exercises and activities like Pilates and dynamic mobility training help prevent stiffness, improve joint health, and support muscle recovery, reducing pain and inflammation in the long term.

Combining these activities ensures your body remains strong, supple, and resilient against chronic inflammation.

4.3 Movement Guidelines: How Much is Enough?

The World Health Organization (WHO)recommends that adults engage in at least:

☐ 150-300minutes of moderate-intensity exercise per week (e.g., brisk walking, cycling)OR

☐ 75-150minutes of vigorous-intensity exercise per week (e.g., running, HIIT workouts).

Additional benefits include two weekly strength training sessions focusing on major muscle groups. If time is limited, even small bursts of movement throughout the day – such as taking the stairs instead of the elevator, doing a few minutes of stretching during work breaks, or standing while working – can provide meaningful health benefits.

Low-impact activities like swimming, chair yoga, or Tai Chi can provide gentle yet effective movement for those with mobility concerns or chronic pain. These activities prove that there's exercise for every body type and ability.

4.4. Real-Life Transformations: How Movement Changed Lives

The impact of exercise is best understood through authentic experiences. Meet Karan and Yasmin, two individuals who transformed their health through movement.

Karan's Story – Overcoming Arthritis with Daily Walks

Karan, a 58-year-old retiree, struggled with arthritis for years. He often felt trapped in his own body, avoiding outings with friends and dreading simple tasks like climbing stairs. His knees ached, his joints felt stiff, and he found himself relying on pain medication to get through the day.

Yasmin's Story – Beating Fatigue with Daily Jogging

Yasmin, a 45-year-old teacher, felt constantly exhausted despite eating well and getting enough sleep. She found herself struggling to focus at work and felt drained even after a full night's sleep. She decided to experiment with morning jogging, starting with just

5-minute runs. Within weeks, she noticed increased energy, mental clarity, and an overall boost in mood. The difference was so profound that she made it a permanent part of her lifestyle. She no longer relies on multiple cups of coffee to stay alert – movement is her natural energy.

These stories highlight a simple truth: regular movement doesn't just improve health, it transforms lives. It inspires, motivates, and shows that change is possible. These stories are a testament to the transformative power of movement and can be the spark that ignites your health journey.

4.5. Family Fitness: Fun & Inclusive Routines

Movement doesn't have to be a solo journey. Involving your family in physical activities fosters healthy habits and strengthens relationships, making you feel connected and part of a supportive community. It's not just about exercise but the shared laughter, the sense of togetherness, and the memories you create.

- Weekend Hikes & Outdoor Adventures: Hiking trails together encourage fitness and create bonding experiences in nature.
- Home Sports Days: Organizing family-friendly competitions (football, basketball, or even backyard obstacle courses) adds a playful element to exercise.
- Active Commuting: Walking or cycling to school/work turns travel time into fitness.
- Evening Walks: A simple stroll after dinner promotes digestion and offers a chance to unwind together.
- Indoor Dance Parties: Turning up the music and dancing in the living room provides an easy, joyful way to stay active.

Interactive Challenge:

Try creating a Family Fitness Calendar, tracking weekly activities, and celebrating milestones with fun rewards like a healthy cooking night or a weekend picnic.

Families build a foundation for lifelong health and well-being by integrating movement into daily routines, intentional movement, deep breathing, and mental relaxation physical resilience and emotional well-being.

4.6. Exploring Mindful Movement

While structured exercise provides powerful anti-inflammatory benefits, another aspect of movement plays a crucial role in holistic health – mindful movement. Yoga and Tai Chi strengthen the body, calm the nervous system, reduce stress hormones, and improve flexibility and balance.

Next, we'll explore how mind-body exercises like yoga, Tai Chi, and mindful movement techniques enhance overall wellness, moving not just a tool for fitness but a practice for mental and emotional health.

4.7. Mindful Movement: Integrating Yoga and Tai Chi for Wellness

Imagine stepping onto a yoga mat and feeling the incredible texture beneath your feet as you take a deep breath. Or picture yourself in a quiet park, gracefully moving through a Tai Chi sequence, each motion flowing like water. These are not just exercises – they are meditative practices that bridge the gap between movement and mindfulness. Unlike high-impact workouts, yoga and Tai Chi blend physical activity with deep breathing, relaxation, and stress reduction, making them powerful tools for combating inflammation and restoring balance to both body and mind.

4.8. How Mindful Movement Supports Anti-Inflammation

Mindful movement focuses on deliberate, controlled actions that engage both the body and the mind. It's a different approach to fitness—one that reduces cortisol levels, regulates inflammatory responses, and promotes overall well-being.

- Yoga: Stress Reduction & Flexibility Yoga is more than just stretching – it's a practice that combines physical postures (asanas), controlled breathing(pranayama), and meditation. Research shows that yoga lowers cortisol (the stress hormone), reduces inflammatory markers, and enhances immune function. Whether you hold a gentle child's pose or flow through sun salutations, each movement helps relieve tension, improve circulation, and promote relaxation.

- Tai Chi: Balance & Joint Health Often described as "meditation in motion," Tai Chi consists of slow, deliberate movements that enhance coordination, strengthen muscles, and improve balance. Its gentle yet consistent movements reduce joint stiffness and improve mobility, making it ideal for people with arthritis or chronic pain.

Both yoga and Tai Chi focus on breath awareness and mindful movement, which help lower inflammation and regulate the nervous system, which are crucial factors in reducing stress-related inflammation.

4.9. Simple Ways to Integrate Mindful Movement into Daily Life

Mindful movement does not require an hour-long session. Even a few minutes each day can have a profound impact.

- Start Small – Try five minutes of gentle stretching or a simple breathing exercise before bed.
- Incorporate Movement Breaks – A few yoga poses, or Tai Chi moves in the morning can help energize the body for the day ahead.
- Mindful Walking – Pay attention to each step, the rhythm of your breath, and the movement of your body. This turns an ordinary walk into a meditative experience.
- Breathe with Intention – Whether seated at your desk or standing in a queue, practice deep, controlled breathing to calm the nervous system and reduce stress.

By weaving these practices into daily life, movement becomes a tool for physical fitness, mental clarity, and inner peace.

4.10. Overcoming Barriers: Making Time for Movement in a Busy Life

Despite knowing the benefits of exercise, many struggle to fit it into their schedules. Lack of time, motivation, and competing responsibilities often stand in the way. But moving as a part of daily life doesn't have to be complicated or time-consuming.

Tackling Common Obstacles to Regular Exercise

- "I don't have time." Instead of setting aside an hour, break exercise into smaller chunks throughout the day. A 10-minute walk in the morning, afternoon stretching, and evening light resistance exercises all add up.
- "I don't enjoy exercise." Find something you love – dancing, cycling, yoga, or hiking. When movement is enjoyable, it becomes a habit rather than a chore.
- "I don't know where to start." Begin with simple activities like walking, body-weight exercises, or yoga. Fitness apps and YouTube workouts can guide you without gym membership.

- "I lack motivation." Set realistic goals and track progress. Aiming for 5,000 steps daily, completing a weekly yoga session, or improving flexibility gives tangible milestones to celebrate.
- "I feel too tired." Ironically, movement boosts energy levels. A short burst of exercise increases blood circulation, releases endorphins, and combats fatigue. The key is to start small and build gradually.

4.11. The Role of Technology & Community in Staying Active

Movement becomes more enjoyable and sustainable when done with others. Joining a walking group, virtual fitness challenge, or local sports club can increase motivation, provide social support, and make exercise feel less like a chore. Fitness apps and wearable trackers can also help by tracking progress, setting reminders, and celebrating milestones, reinforcing positive movement habits.

Modern tools make it easier to stay on track with fitness goals.

- Fitness Apps & Trackers – Devices like Fitbits and smartwatches monitor steps, heart rate, and activity levels, keeping you accountable.
- Online Workout Classes – Virtual sessions in yoga, HIIT, or Pilates allow you to work out from home.
- Community Support – Engaging in group fitness challenges or joining local walking groups adds social motivation to movement.

By leveraging technology and social support, staying active becomes easier and more enjoyable.

4.12. Prioritising Movement: A Commitment to Lifelong Health

At the heart of this journey lies a simple truth: movement is not a luxury, it's essential for long-term health. By overcoming barriers and incorporating exercise into daily life, you take charge of your well-being in a way that no medication can replicate.

- ☐ Small, consistent efforts are more impactful than occasional intense workouts.
- ☐ Prioritizing movement is a mindset shift – treat exercise as a non-negotiable part of self-care.
- ☐ Find joy in movement through dance, yoga, walking, or sports.

Incorporating movement doesn't just add years to your life, it adds quality to those years.

Closing Thoughts & Transition to Chapter 4

As we conclude this chapter, remember that movement is a powerful, accessible medicine that strengthens the body, sharpens the mind, and supports overall well-being.

Your Healing Reflection:

- How do you feel after movement or exercise – physically and mentally?
- What would it take to make regular movement a joyful habit in your life?

Please complete the 'I will ...' statement on page 5.

Chapter Five

SPICES ARE MEDICINE

Unlocking the Healing Power of Nature's Flavors

The History of Spices as Medicine

For thousands of years, spices have been valued not only for their ability to enhance flavor but also for their medicinal properties. Long before modern pharmaceuticals, ancient civilizations recognized the healing power of spices, using them to treat ailments, boost immunity, and preserve food. Traditional medical systems such as Ayurveda in India, Traditional Chinese Medicine, and Arabic Unani medicine incorporated spices like turmeric, cinnamon, and black pepper as essential tools for maintaining health and preventing disease.

The demand for these potent ingredients set the stage for one of the most influential economic movements in history – the spice trade. European explorers, fascinated by the exotic spices of the Middle East, India, and China, embarked on perilous voyages in search of direct trade routes. The Portuguese, Dutch, and British empires all competed fiercely to control the spice trade, establishing colonies and influencing global commerce for centuries. Spices became as valuable as gold, fuelling economic expansion and shaping the course of world history.

Christianne, a researcher studying the medicinal properties of spices, is uncovering how these ancient ingredients hold scientific merit beyond folklore. Today, modern science is rediscovering what ancient cultures have long known – spices are powerful natural medicines. Research continues to confirm their anti-inflammatory, antimicrobial, and antioxidant properties, reinforcing their role in disease prevention and holistic healing.

5.1 Introduction to Spices: Natural Remedies for Inflammation:

Imagine yourself in a bustling spice market, surrounded by a kaleidoscope of vibrant colors and intoxicating aromas. Each stall is a treasure trove of exotic spices, waiting to be discovered. These are not just ingredients to flavor your meals; they are potent tools in your health arsenal. As you explore the myriad choices, consider the potential of each spice in combating inflammation, a common challenge as we navigate the transitions of middle age. Spices like turmeric, chili peppers, cinnamon, and coriander offer a natural, flavorful approach to managing inflammation, turning your kitchen into a hub of health enhancement and culinary delight.

5.2 The Science Behind Spices' Anti-Inflammatory Power

At the heart of many spices' anti-inflammatory properties lies their ability to influence inflammation at a molecular level. Take turmeric, for instance. Its active compound, curcumin, plays a crucial role in inhibiting NF-kB, a protein complex that drives inflammatory responses in the body. By blocking this pathway, curcumin reduces the production of pro-inflammatory molecules, offering relief from conditions that thrive on chronic inflammation. Imagine adding a dash of turmeric to your morning smoothie or evening curry, knowing it's actively working to soothe inflammation from within.

Chili peppers, too, wield impressive anti-inflammatory power through capsaicin, their fiery component. Capsaicin reduces substance P levels, a neuropeptide involved in transmitting pain and inflammation signals. This reduction can alleviate symptoms associated with neurogenic inflammation, such as joint pain and swelling. Picture the vibrant red of chili peppers enhancing your favorite dish, not just with heat but with health benefits that resonate throughout your body.

The antioxidant properties of spices further amplify their role in combating inflammation. Spices like cinnamon are rich in polyphenols, which neutralize free radicals and reduce oxidative stress – a key contributor to inflammation. Sprinkle cinnamon over your oatmeal or into a warm beverage to add warmth and sweetness and fortify your body's defenses against cellular damage. Similarly, the flavonoids in coriander offer protection by shielding cells from oxidative harm, helping maintain cellular integrity and function.

5.3 Mental Health and Spices

Spices not only enhance physical health but also play a profound role in mental well-being. Chronic inflammation has been linked to a variety of mental health issues, including depression, anxiety, and cognitive decline. By incorporating anti-inflammatory spices into your diet, you can help reduce inflammation and support a healthier mind, a lesser known but significant benefit of these powerful ingredients.

Turmeric, with its active compound curcumin, has been shown to have antidepressant-like effects. Several studies indicate that curcumin can help reduce symptoms of depression by boosting levels of serotonin and dopamine in the brain, neurotransmitters critical for mood regulation. This makes turmeric a powerful ally in physical inflammation and addresses the psychological effects of chronic inflammation.

Similarly, ginger has been studied for its anti-anxiety effects, with research showing that it can help reduce anxiety symptoms and improve cognitive function. Ginger is rich in antioxidants, which protect the brain from oxidative stress, one of the underlying causes of neurodegeneration. This makes ginger a valuable addition to a diet that supports mental and physical health.

Cinnamon, another spice with well-documented health benefits, has also been linked to improved cognitive function. Studies have shown that the polyphenols in cinnamon can help reduce brain inflammation, potentially boosting memory and focus. Adding cinnamon to your morning oatmeal or incorporating it into your drinks can boost your mental clarity, making it an excellent spice for mood and brain health.

5.4 The Role of Indian Spices in Healing

Indian spices have long been revered for their therapeutic properties, deeply rooted in the rich traditions of Ayurveda. The use of spices like turmeric, cardamom, ginger, and fenugreek in Indian cuisine is integral to maintaining health and wellness. For instance, turmeric (often paired with black pepper for better absorption) is a staple in cooking and traditional remedies to treat inflammation and boost immunity. Cardamom and ginger are known for their digestive benefits, helping reduce bloating and supporting the body's detoxification processes. Additionally, fenugreek is widely used in Indian cooking to regulate blood sugar levels and manage diabetes-related inflammation.

These spices provide essential health benefits beyond just flavoring food, aligning with holistic health practices. They can significantly reduce the risk of chronic inflammatory diseases and enhance general well-being, offering a natural and effective way to balance your body's systems.

5.5 Scientific Validation of Spices' Health Claims

Scientific studies have increasingly supported the health claims of spices, validating their traditional uses with modern evidence. Research on ginger, for instance, has demonstrated its ability to reduce muscle pain and inflammation, highlighting its potential as a natural remedy for exercise-induced discomfort. Incorporating ginger into your diet can be as simple as adding fresh slices to tea or grating it into stir-fries, each bite offering a dose of natural relief. Meanwhile, black pepper's active compound, piperine, enhances the absorption of curcumin, making it a valuable companion to turmeric. This synergistic relationship underscores the importance of combining spices for maximum health benefits, providing you with a solid scientific foundation to trust in the power of spices.

5.6 Integrating Spices into Your Daily Routine

Integrating spices into your daily routine offers a dual advantage: they elevate the flavor of your meals while promoting better health. Imagine transforming a simple chicken dish with a blend of spices that tantalizes your taste buds and contributes to your well-being. Spices make healthy foods palatable, encouraging you to enjoy a diverse and nutritious diet. By embracing the flavorful world of spices, you enhance your culinary experiences and health, discovering that the path to wellness can be as delicious as beneficial.

5.7 Spice Integration Checklist

- ☐ Turmeric: Add to soups, smoothies, and curries for anti-inflammatory benefits.
    - ☐ Chili Peppers: Use in stews and sauces to reduce pain and inflammation.
    - ☐ Cinnamon: Sprinkle on oats and in drinks for antioxidant effects.
    - ☐ Coriander: Incorporate into salads and marinades for cellular protection.

☐ Black Pepper: Pair with turmeric to boost curcumin absorption.

5.8 Essential Spice Guide: Flavor Profiles and Health Benefits

As you explore the colorful world of spices, imagine each one as a small, potent ally in your quest for better health. Turmeric's earthy flavor is famous for its anti-inflammatory and antioxidant properties. Known as the "golden spice," it adds a warm, vibrant hue to your dishes while supporting your body's defenses. Its versatility means you can sprinkle it into soups, stews, or rice dishes, transforming them into health-boosting meals.

With its sweet and woody aroma, Cinnamon offers more than just flavor. It plays a significant role in regulating blood sugar levels, making it a valuable addition to your diet, especially if you manage your glucose. Consider adding a dash of cinnamon to your morning coffee or oatmeal, turning these everyday staples into health-enhancing treats. The comforting scent of cinnamon can evoke a sense of warmth and nostalgia, making your meals both delicious and beneficial.

Cardamom, with its citrus-like flavor, aids digestion and can help reduce bloating. This spice is often used in sweet and savory dishes, lending its unique taste to both. You might include cardamom in baked goods like cookies or cakes or savory dishes like curries and stews. Its ability to support digestive health makes it a perfect ingredient for those who experience occasional digestive discomfort, offering relief with every bite.

Pairing spices with different foods can maximize their health benefits and elevate your culinary creations. Ginger, for instance, pairs beautifully with fish dishes. Its zesty kick not only enhances the flavor of the fish but also aids digestion. Imagine a fresh salmon fillet marinated with ginger, garlic, and a splash of lemon juice, baked to perfection. This combination delights the palate and supports your digestive health, making each meal a nourishing experience.

Cumin is another spice that can transform your meals with its warm, earthy notes. It's particularly effective in legume recipes like lentil soups or chickpea stews. Cumin not only boosts the flavor of these dishes but also aids in nutrient absorption, ensuring you get the most out of your meals. Its ability to enhance taste and nutrition makes cumin a staple in many kitchens, offering a simple way to improve your diet.

The cultural significance of spices adds another layer to their use. Saffron, known for its rich color and subtle flavor, is a prized ingredient in Middle Eastern cuisine. Often used in dishes like paella or risotto, saffron brings visual appeal and health benefits and is known for its potential for mood enhancement and antioxidant properties. Similarly, curry leaves are a staple in Indian cooking, traditionally used to support digestion. When added to soups or stews, these leaves impart a distinct flavor that speaks to their cultural roots.

5.9 Cooking with Spices: Easy Recipes to Boost Health

Imagine a chilly evening where all you crave is a comforting, warm beverage that delights your senses and nourishes your body. The Golden Turmeric Latte is just that – a soothing drink rich in anti-inflammatory properties, making it a perfect choice to unwind. To prepare this, start by warming a cup of milk, whether dairy or a plant-based alternative, over medium heat. Whisk in a teaspoon of turmeric powder, a pinch of black pepper, and a hint of cinnamon as it simmers. Add a teaspoon of honey or maple syrup to taste. Stir until everything is well combined and frothy. Pour the latte into your favorite mug and enjoy this golden elixir that warms you up and supports your body's natural defenses against inflammation.

For a more substantial meal, consider a Spiced Quinoa Salad, a dish that combines the nutty flavor of quinoa with the vibrant cumin, coriander, and lemon spices. Start by cooking one cup of quinoa per the instructions, then let it cool. Mix the quinoa with a handful of chopped parsley, diced cucumber, and cherry tomatoes in a large bowl. For the dressing, whisk together the juice of one lemon with a teaspoon of ground cumin and coriander, a pinch of salt, and a drizzle of olive oil. Toss the salad with the dressing, adjusting the spices to your preference. With its refreshing crunch and zest, this salad is not only delicious but also packed with nutrients that support digestion and overall health.

Maximizing spices' flavor and health benefits requires specific techniques, such as tempering. This involves briefly frying spices in oil, which releases their essential oils and enhances their flavors. When you prepare curry or stew, start by heating a tablespoon of oil in a pan. Add whole spices like cumin or mustard seeds, allowing them to sizzle and pop for a few seconds before adding the other ingredients. This simple step can transform a dish, enriching it with deeper flavors and making the spices more effective in supporting health.

Another method to enhance the depth of flavor and health benefits of spices is to infuse them in broths. Whether you're making a soup or a stew, add whole spices like bay leaves or cloves to the simmering broth. The slow cooking process allows the spices to release their flavors gradually, creating a rich and aromatic base for your dish. This technique not only elevates the taste but also ensures that the health-promoting properties of the spices are fully integrated into the meal.

Proper storage is crucial to maintain the potency and freshness of your spices. Keep them in airtight containers (not plastic) to protect them from exposure to air, which can cause them to lose their flavor and effectiveness. Store these containers in a cool, dark place, away from heat and light, which can degrade the quality of the spices overtime. By taking these simple precautions, you ensure that your spices remain a potent ally in your culinary and health endeavors, ready to enhance your dishes whenever needed.

5.10 Global Flavors: Incorporating Ethnic Spices into Your Diet

Imagine stepping into a kitchen where the world's flavors come alive, each spice telling its own story. You pick up a jar of za'atar, a mesmerizing blend of thyme, sumac, and sesame seeds. This Middle Eastern staple offers a nutty and tangy profile that effortlessly elevates breads and roasted vegetables. Picture a warm flatbread drizzled with olive oil, sprinkled generously with za'atar, and baked until crisp. This simple yet flavorful dish invites you to explore the rich culinary traditions of the Levant, where meals are often a communal celebration of flavor and fellowship.

Turn your gaze toward North Africa, where the fiery allure of harissa awaits. This spicy chili paste, infused with garlic and caraway, packs a punch that ignites the senses. It's the secret behind many Moroccan stews, adding depth and heat to every bite. Consider using harissa as a marinade for grilled meats or stirring it into soups for an invigorating kick. Its boldness encourages you to embrace the vibrant, spice-forward dishes of North Africa, inviting you to savor the heat and complexity that harissa brings to the table.

Ethnic spices like sumac and fenugreek offer flavor and health benefits. With its tart, lemony notes, sumac is a powerhouse of antioxidants, helping to reduce oxidative stress. A dash of sumac over a salad or grilled chicken adds brightness and a healthful edge. Fenugreek, often used in Indian and Middle Eastern cooking, plays a role in blood sugar control. Its slightly bitter, maple-like flavor can be found in curries and spice blends. These spices enhance your meals and support well-being, bridging the gap between culinary delight and health.

Conclusion: Cooking with Spices for Health and Wellness

By incorporating these ethnic spices into your diet, you not only enhance flavor but also embrace centuries of healing wisdom. Christianne, a researcher studying the medicinal properties of spices, has uncovered how cultures worldwide have long understood their power in promoting health. Today, modern science is catching up, proving that spices possess anti-inflammatory, antimicrobial, and antioxidant properties that contribute to disease prevention and holistic well-being.

Each meal invites us to explore, learn, and appreciate the diverse flavors that unite us all. These spices remind us that food is a universal language that speaks of heritage, health, and harmony. As you continue experimenting and enjoying these global flavors, remember that each spice is a bridge to understanding and a celebration of our shared human experience.

Your journey toward health is not just personal – it is connected to traditions, communities, and global well-being. With every spice you use and every dish you prepare, you participate in a larger movement that honors the past while nourishing the future. The best time to start is now.

Your Healing Reflection:

- What spices do you already use?

- Which healing spices from this chapter are you curious to try more regularly in your meals?

Please complete the 'I will ...' statement on page 5.

Chapter Six

Mental Health & Whole-Body Well-Being

Nurturing the Mind for a Healthier Body and Spirit

"We are facing an unprecedented mental health crisis. Social pressures, economic uncertainty, digital overload, and lifestyle changes have fuelled a sharp rise in anxiety, depression, and burnout. While awareness has improved, stigma remains a major barrier, and healthcare systems are struggling to keep up." This insight from a leading consultant psychiatrist highlight the growing burden of mental illness. Today's world is overwhelming, with chronic stress, poor diet, sleep deprivation, and reduced social connections creating an environment where mental well-being is constantly under strain.

Mental health is not just a brain issue – it affects the entire body. Inês, a dedicated mental health nurse, has seen first hand how emotional struggles manifest physically, from chronic pain to digestive issues and fatigue. Addressing mental health requires more than just medication and therapy – it calls for a whole-body approach. Nutrition, sleep, movement, and social engagement are all essential for restoring emotional balance and resilience.

By shifting the conversation to prevention and holistic healing, we can create a healthier foundation for mental well-being. Mental health is not just about the mind. It reveals itself through posture, tension, breath, digestion, and silent strain. The emotional burden is woven through the entire body. Inês works with her patients to integrate simple, sustainable habits - ensuring that mental wellness is supported through treatment and everyday lifestyle choices. Her experience highlights that true healing is found in the mind, body, and community connection.

6.1 Introduction: Mental Health & Whole-Body Well-Being

Mental health is deeply interconnected with nutrition, gut health, inflammation, and lifestyle choices. While mental well-being has traditionally been viewed through a psychological lens, emerging research highlights the decisive role of diet, movement, and gut-brain communication in emotional resilience and cognitive function. The brain does not operate in isolation; it is constantly influenced by systemic inflammation, nutrient availability, and gut microbiome health. Chronic stress, poor diet, and lack of movement can exacerbate neuroinflammation, disrupting neurotransmitter balance and contributing to conditions like anxiety, depression, and cognitive decline. By making strategic dietary and lifestyle changes, we can support neurotransmitter production, reduce brain inflammation, and improve mental clarity and emotional stability.

6.2 The Gut-Brain Axis: The Missing Link in Mental Health

Have you ever had a "gut feeling" about something? It turns out that's more than just a saying – the gut and brain are in constant communication. This gut-brain axis is a two-way communication network linking the central nervous system (CNS) and the gut microbiome, playing a key role in mood regulation, cognitive function, and emotional resilience.

Your gut is home to trillions of bacteria, and many of them produce neurotransmitters that directly impact your mental health:

☐ Serotonin – The Happiness Chemical

Around 90% of your body's serotonin – a neurotransmitter responsible for mood, sleep, and emotional stability – is produced in the gut. Beneficial bacteria convert dietary tryptophan (found in turkey, eggs, nuts, and seeds) into serotonin, helping to regulate mood. When the gut microbiome is imbalanced, serotonin production can drop, leading to low mood, anxiety, and poor stress response.

☐ Dopamine – The Motivation & Reward Neurotransmitter

Dopamine is responsible for pleasure, motivation, and focus. Certain gut bacteria, such as Lactobacillus plantarum and Bifidobacterium infantis, influence dopamine synthesis. A disrupted gut microbiome can reduce dopamine levels, leading to brain fog, lack of motivation, and difficulty experiencing joy.

- GABA – The Brain's Natural Relaxant

GABA(gamma-aminobutyric acid) is a calming neurotransmitter that helps you manage stress and anxiety. Specific probiotic strains, like Bifidobacterium and Lactobacillus, can naturally enhance GABA production, promoting relaxation and better sleep.

If your gut microbiome is out of balance – due to stress, processed foods, excessive sugar, or antibiotic overuse – it can reduce neurotransmitter production, affecting mental clarity, focus, and emotional stability.

6.3 How Inflammation Affects Your Brain

You might associate inflammation with a swollen ankle or a sore throat, but did you know it can silently impact your brain, too? Chronic, low-grade inflammation is now recognized as a major driver of mental health disorders, including anxiety, depression, and cognitive decline.

The body releases pro-inflammatory molecules called cytokines when it experiences ongoing stress, poor diet, or gut imbalances. These cytokines can cross the blood-brain barrier, triggering neuroinflammation linked to brain fog, mood instability, and impaired focus.

Here's how chronic inflammation affects your brain:

- Disrupts Neurotransmitter Balance – Inflammation reduces serotonin and dopamine levels, contributing to low mood, irritability, and loss of motivation.
- Increases Cortisol (The Stress Hormone) – Prolonged stress and inflammation keep cortisol levels high, leading to fatigue, anxiety, and trouble sleeping.
- Damages Brain Cells –Inflammatory molecules like TNF-alpha and IL-6 can accelerate oxidative stress, damaging neurons and increasing the risk of cognitive decline and memory loss.

If left unchecked, chronic inflammation weakens the gut-brain connection, making the brain more vulnerable to stress, anxiety, and depression. The good news? By reducing inflammation through diet, lifestyle, and stress management, you can protect your brain and boost your mental resilience.

Try This: Reduce brain inflammation by adding anti-inflammatory foods like turmeric, leafy greens, fatty fish, and extra virgin olive oil to your diet. These foods help regulate cytokine activity, supporting cognitive health and emotional balance.

Try This: To keep your gut-brain axis strong, focus on gut-friendly foods like fermented foods(yogurt, kimchi, kefir), prebiotics (onions, garlic, bananas), and polyphenol-rich foods (berries, green tea, dark chocolate).

6.4 Brain-Boosting Nutrients: What to Eat for Mental Clarity & Emotional Balance

Your brain is an energy-demanding powerhouse, constantly working to process information, regulate emotions, and support memory. To function at its best, it needs the proper nutrients – and the foods you eat directly affect neurotransmitter balance, stress resilience, and mental performance.

Here are some of the top brain-boosting nutrients and how they support your mental health:

- Omega-3 Fatty Acids: Cognitive Performance & Synaptic Plasticity

  Why it matters: Omega-3s – especially DHA (docosahexaenoic acid) and EPA (eicosapentaenoic acid) – are critical for brain structure and function.

  How it helps: DHA supports neuronal flexibility and communication, while EPA reduces neuroinflammation, lowering the risk of depression and cognitive decline.

  Where to get it: Fatty fish (salmon, sardines, mackerel), flaxseeds, chia seeds, walnuts, algae-based DHA supplements.

- Polyphenols: Anti-Aging & Brain Protection

  Why it matters: These powerful antioxidants protect neurons from oxidative stress and inflammation, two major drivers of brain aging and mood disorders.

  How it helps: Polyphenols boost BDNF (brain-derived neurotrophic factor), a protein that enhances memory, learning, and neuroprotection.

Where to get it: Blueberries, blackberries, dark chocolate (85% cocoa), extra virgin olive oil, green tea, turmeric.

- Choline: The Memory & Focus Nutrient

Why it matters: Choline is a precursor to acetylcholine, a neurotransmitter essential for memory formation, learning, and focus.

How it helps: It improves synaptic signaling and supports long-term cognitive health.

Where to get it: Eggs, fatty fish, beef liver, soybeans, broccoli, Brussels sprouts.

- Zinc & Magnesium: Stress Resilience & Emotional Stability

Why they matter: Zinc and magnesium regulate stress hormones, improve emotional stability, and enhance neurotransmitter function.

- How they help:

Zinc plays a role in neuroplasticity, learning, and mood regulation - a deficiency is linked to anxiety and depression.

Magnesium is a relaxation mineral that helps reduce cortisol, promote better sleep, and support brain health.

- Where to get them: Nuts (almonds, cashews), seeds (pumpkin seeds, sunflower seeds), leafy greens, dark chocolate, whole grains.

Your diet directly influences mental health, and by including these key brain-boosting nutrients, you can enhance mood stability, memory, and overall cognitive function.

Try This: Eat at least three of these brain-supporting foods daily to optimize your mental clarity and emotional well-being.

6.5 The Power of Food: How Your Diet Impacts Mental Health

It's easy to overlook the role of food unemotional well-being, but your diet is one of the most powerful tools for supporting mental resilience. The nutrients you consume influence neurotransmitter production, stress response, and inflammation levels, all affecting mood and cognition.

Let's break it down:
Blood Sugar Balance & Mood Stability

- Why it matters: Fluctuations in blood sugar levels can cause energy crashes, mood swings, and irritability.

- How to stabilize it: Choose complex carbohydrates (quinoa, oats, sweet potatoes) overrefined sugars to maintain steady energy and focus.

Gut Health & Emotional Regulation

- Why it matters: A healthy gut microbiome produces neurotransmitters and regulates inflammation, directly impacting stress levels and emotional stability.
- How to support it: Include fermented foods (yogurt, kimchi, sauerkraut), prebiotic fibers (garlic, onions, asparagus), and polyphenol-rich foods (berries, green tea, dark chocolate).

Inflammation & Cognitive Performance

- Why it matters: Chronic inflammation is linked to brain fog, memory loss, and increased anxiety or depression.
- How to reduce it: Eat anti-inflammatory foods like fatty fish, turmeric, extra virgin olive oil, leafy greens, and nuts while avoiding processed and ultra-processed foods that fuel inflammation.

Try This:

- Make one meal daily rich in brain-boosting foods like Omega-3s, fiber, and polyphenols.
- Swap sugary snacks for mood-friendly options like nuts, dark chocolate, or probiotic yogurt.
- Plan meals with stable blood sugar in mind – combine protein, healthy fats, and fiber to avoid crashes.

Fuelling your brain with the right nutrients can improve focus, emotional resilience, and long-term mental health.

6.6 The Role of Movement in Mental Health: Why Exercise is Essential

Did you know that regular movement is one of the most effective natural antidepressants? Exercise doesn't just strengthen your muscles—it also enhances brain function, reduces stress, and improves mood stability.

- Increases BDNF (Brain-Derived Neurotrophic Factor): Exercise boosts BDNF levels, which support memory formation, learning, and neuroplasticity.
- Enhances Neurotransmitter Production: Movement increases dopamine, serotonin, and endorphins, naturally lifting mood and reducing anxiety.

- Reduces Cortisol & Inflammation: Exercise lowers chronic stress hormones, helping to calm the nervous system and improve resilience to daily stressors.
- Strengthens Gut-Brain Communication: Studies show that regular physical activity improves gut microbial diversity and positively affects mental well-being.

Best Forms of Exercise for Mental Well-Being

Aerobic Exercise (Walking, Running, Cycling, Swimming)

- Boosts oxygen flow to the brain, improving focus & clarity.
- Reduces cortisol levels, promoting emotional resilience.
- Encourages the release of endorphins, which naturally combat stress & depression.

Strength Training (Bodyweight, Resistance Bands, Weightlifting)

- Helps regulate neurotransmitters & stress hormones.
- Increases testosterone & growth hormones, protecting against brain aging.
- Improves insulin sensitivity, stabilizing mood and energy.

Yoga, Tai Chi & Stretching

- Activates the parasympathetic nervous system, reducing stress & promoting relaxation.
- Improves body awareness & mind-body connection, helping ease anxiety.
- Increases GABA production, supporting better sleep & mood balance.

Try This:

- Incorporate 30-45 minutes of movement daily – whether it's a brisk walk, weight training, or stretching.
- Get outdoors. Sunlight exposure during exercise enhances Vitamin D production, improving mood.
- If you're anxious, try 10 minutes of deep breathing, yoga, or gentle movement to reset your nervous system.

When you move your body, you heal your mind. Making exercise a consistent part of your routine can reduce stress, enhance brain function, and build long-term emotional resilience.

6.7 Stress Management: Training Your Brain to Stay Resilient

Stress is unavoidable, but how you respond can transform your mental well-being. Chronic stress keeps your cortisol levels elevated, which can lead to anxiety, burnout, sleep issues, and even memory loss. The good news? There are powerful, science-backed techniques that can rewire your brain to handle stress more effectively.

The Science of Stress & Cortisol Regulation

- Cortisol, the stress hormone, is helpful in small doses – it sharpens focus and boosts alertness.
- Chronic stress elevates cortisol, leading to brain fog, inflammation, and mood swings.
- Stress resilience isn't about avoiding stress – it's about training your body to recover quickly.

Stress-Busting Techniques That Work

Mindfulness & Meditation

- Trains the brain to stay present, reducing stress reactivity.
- Strengthens the prefrontal cortex, which helps with emotional regulation.
- Lowers amygdala overactivity – the brain region responsible for fear and anxiety.

Breathwork for Nervous System Balance

- Box Breathing (4-4-4-4 count): Activates the parasympathetic nervous system, calming stress.
- Alternate Nostril Breathing: Synchronizes brain hemispheres, improving focus.
- Diaphragmatic Breathing: Slows heart rate & reduces inflammatory markers in the bloodstream.

Nature Therapy & Grounding

- Exposure to green spaces reduces cortisol & boosts dopamine production.
- Walking barefoot on natural surfaces (grass, sand) enhances vagus nerve activation, improving stress resilience.
- Just 20 minutes outdoors can significantly lower stress levels.

Creative Outlets: Music, Writing & Art Therapy

- Engaging in creative activities stimulates neural pathways linked to joy & emotional processing.
- Playing music or writing increases dopamine, improving motivation and mental clarity.

Try This:

- Practice deep breathing five minutes before meals to activate your "rest-and-digest" system, which will improve gut health and relaxation.
- Schedule 10–20 minutes of mindfulness or meditation daily to rewire your brain for emotional balance.

- Spend at least 20 minutes outdoors daily – whether walking, sitting in the sun, or practicing grounding techniques.

Stress may be inevitable, but how you manage it determines its impact on your mental health. You can build resilience and maintain emotional well-being by training your brain and body to reset quickly.

6.8 Global Meal Plan for Mental Health

Eating for mental health is about balance, diversity, and nutrient density. The following meals incorporate traditional ingredients from various global cuisines, each offering anti-inflammatory benefits, neurotransmitter support, and gut-health-boosting properties.

Breakfast: Energy & Mental Clarity

Indian Spiced Moong Dal Chilla (Savory Lentil Pancakes) with Yogurt & Mint Chutney

- Lentils provide prebiotic fiber – Supports gut microbiome & serotonin production.
- Turmeric & cumin reduce inflammation – Enhances cognitive function.
- Yogurt provides probiotics – Supports gut-brain axis & emotional balance.

Vietnamese Pho-Inspired Breakfast Broth with Tofu & Mushrooms

- Rich in umami compounds – Enhances dopamine levels.
- Mushrooms support nerve regeneration – Contain neuroprotective compounds.
- Cinnamon & star anise regulate blood sugar – Stabilizes energy & mood.

Lunch: Mental Clarity & Mood Stability

Mexican Black Bean & Avocado Tostadas with Fermented Salsa

- Black beans provide folate & magnesium – Key for stress regulation.
- Fermented salsa (with pickled onions & garlic) – Boosts gut diversity.
- Avocado provides healthy fats – Supports dopamine & serotonin production.

Japanese Miso & Seaweed Soup with Fermented Tofu & Brown Rice

- Miso contains probiotics – Enhances gut-brain axis & serotonin levels.
- Seaweed provides iodine & omega-3s – Supports brain function.
- Brown rice offers magnesium & B vitamins – Supports stress resilience.

Dinner: Neuroprotection & Emotional Balance

Thai Green Curry with Coconut Milk, Lemongrass & Tofu

- ☐ Coconut milk contains healthy fats – Essential for brain function.
- ☐ Galangal & lemongrass are rich in antioxidants – Reduce neuroinflammation.
- ☐ Tofu provides plant-based proteins – Aid in neurotransmitter production.

Mediterranean Chickpea & Eggplant Stew with Olive Oil & Herbs
- ☐ Rich in polyphenols from extra virgin olive oil – Protects against brain aging.
- ☐ Chickpeas provide prebiotics – Promote gut health & mood stability.
- ☐ Rosemary & thyme improve cognitive function – Boost memory & focus.

Evening Snack: Optimizing Sleep & Relaxation

Korean Fermented Kimchi Pancakes with Sesame Seeds
- ☐ Kimchi provides probiotics – Strengthens gut-brain communication.
- ☐ Sesame seeds contain zinc & magnesium – Support relaxation & deep sleep.

Greek Yogurt with Honey, Walnuts & Pomegranate Seeds
- ☐ Probiotics from yogurt – Enhance serotonin production.
- ☐ Polyphenols from pomegranate – Protect against oxidative stress.
- ☐ Omega-3s from walnuts – Improve cognitive function.

Try This:
- ☐ Experiment with traditional dishes from different cultures – they offer unique nutrient profiles for brain health.
- ☐ Fermented foods (miso, kimchi, yogurt, pickled vegetables) should be part of your daily meals to strengthen gut-brain communication.
- ☐ Rotate plant-based proteins from different cuisines (lentils, tofu, chickpeas, black beans) to support neurotransmitter production.

By embracing global meal diversity, you can fuel your brain with rich flavors while nourishing your gut and mental well-being.

6.9 Checklist for Nutritional Mental Health Support

Building a brain-friendly diet doesn't have to be complicated. Here's a quick checklist to help you integrate key nutrients and lifestyle strategies for optimal mental clarity, emotional balance, and long-term resilience.

- ☐ Prioritize Omega-3s Daily – Include fatty fish (salmon, sardines), walnuts, flaxseeds, or algae-based supplements to reduce inflammation and support neurotransmitter function.
- ☐ Eat Probiotic & Fermented Foods – Consume yogurt, kimchi, miso, kefir, and pickled vegetables to boost gut microbiome diversity and improve serotonin production.

- ☐ Support Gut Health with Prebiotics – Fiber-rich foods like onions, garlic, leeks, asparagus, and bananas feed beneficial gut bacteria, strengthening the gut-brain axis.
- ☐ Include B Vitamins & Magnesium – Eat leafy greens, whole grains, legumes, nuts, and seeds to regulate stress hormones and neurotransmitter production.
- ☐ Limit Ultra-Processed & Sugary Foods – Reduce refined sugars, artificial sweeteners, and highly processed snacks, as they can disrupt gut health and increase inflammation.
- ☐ Opt for Whole, Anti-Inflammatory Foods – Add turmeric, ginger, olive oil, dark leafy greens, and berries to your daily meals to support cognitive health and lower oxidative stress.
- ☐ Balance Blood Sugar – Pair healthy fats, proteins, and fiber in meals to avoid energy crashes, mood swings, and brain fog.
- ☐ Stay Hydrated – Drink sufficient water and herbal teas to maintain cognitive function and prevent fatigue.
- ☐ Monitor Vitamin D Levels – Spend time outdoors or supplement as needed to support mood regulation and immune function.
- ☐ Incorporate Mindful Eating – Slow down, chew thoroughly, and be present while eating to enhance digestion and gut-brain communication.
- ☐ Exercise Regularly – Engage in aerobic movement, strength training, or yoga to boost neurotransmitter levels and reduce stress.
- ☐ Prioritize Sleep – Aim for 7-9 hours of quality sleep to allow the brain to detox, regulate emotions, and enhance cognitive function.

Try This:
- ☐ Start small! Choose and implement one or two changes from the checklist this week.
- ☐ Track how you feel – better energy, improved mood, and reduced stress are signs of progress.
- ☐ Make mental health nutrition part of your lifestyle rather than a short-term fix.

By integrating these simple dietary and lifestyle strategies, you can support long-term brain health, improve focus, and naturally reduce stress.

6.10 Final Thoughts: The Mind-Body Connection

Your mental health isn't just about what's happening in your mind – it's about what's happening in your entire body. Everything is connected to your brain and gut: food, movement, stress levels, and sleep habits. When you nourish your body, you nourish your mind. When you strengthen your gut, you improve your resilience.

Healing doesn't happen overnight, but every small step you take matters. Choosing a brain-boosting meal, stepping outside for a walk, and practicing deep breathing are daily habits that create a foundation for lifelong mental well-being.

Your brain is adaptable. Your body is resilient. Your mental health is within your power. The foods you eat, the way you move, and how you manage stress – these choices influence your mood, focus, and emotional balance. And the best part? You get to take control.

Take the Next Step

- Pick one small change today. Maybe it's adding fermented foods to your diet, prioritizing sleep, or practicing mindfulness.
- Pay attention to how you feel. Notice the shifts – more energy, better focus, improved mood.
- Be patient with yourself. Mental health isn't about perfection – it's about progress.

Remember This:

- Food is medicine – use it to fuel your brain.
- Movement is therapy – let it clear your mind.
- Rest is power – prioritize it for emotional stability.
- You are responsible for your well-being – small steps lead to lasting change.

Your mind and body are on the same team. Take care of them both, and they will take care of you.

6.11 The Role of Spirituality in Mental Well-Being

Mental health is more than physical and emotional – it's also about finding meaning, purpose, and connection. Whether through faith, mindfulness, gratitude, or time in nature, spirituality can reduce stress, enhance resilience, and bring inner peace. Simple practices like deep breathing, meditation, journaling, or engaging in acts of kindness can help quiet the mind, improve emotional balance, and strengthen mental clarity.

6.12 Summary of Key Takeaways: Your Mental Health Roadmap

Your brain, body, and spirit work together, and the choices you make every day shape your mental resilience. Here's what to remember:

Your Gut Health Shapes Your Mental Well-Being
- The gut-brain axis directly links your microbiome and mood regulation.
- Serotonin, dopamine, and GABA – essential neurotransmitters – are influenced by gut bacteria.
- A diverse, well-nourished gut microbiome can improve mood, focus, and emotional balance.
- Try This: Add fermented foods (yogurt, kimchi, kefir) and prebiotics (garlic, onions, fiber-rich veggies) to strengthen gut-brain communication.

Chronic Inflammation Affects Mental Clarity & Mood
- Neuroinflammation contributes to depression, anxiety, and brain fog.
- Sugar, processed foods, and refined oils fuel inflammation, worsening symptoms.
- Anti-inflammatory foods like fatty fish, olive oil, turmeric, and leafy greens help protect the brain.
- Try This: Reduce processed foods and include at least one anti-inflammatory ingredient in every meal.

Nutrients That Support Brain Function & Emotional Balance
- Omega-3s(from salmon, walnuts, flaxseeds) strengthen neurons and improve focus.
- Polyphenols(from berries, dark chocolate, and olive oil) combat brain aging.
- Choline(from eggs, soybeans, fish) boosts memory and cognitive performance.
- Zinc& magnesium (from seeds, nuts, and greens) support neurotransmitter function and stress resilience.
- Try This: Eat various whole, unprocessed foods to give your brain the proper nutrients daily.

Exercise, Stress Management & Spiritual Well-Being Are Essential
- Movement increases BDNF, enhancing memory, learning, and stress tolerance.
- Exercise boosts dopamine, serotonin, and endorphins, naturally lifting mood.

- Breathwork, mindfulness, and spiritual reflection promote resilience and emotional balance.
- Try This: Move for 30-45 minutes daily, practice five minutes of deep breathing, and spend time in self-reflection or gratitude practices.

Sleep & Mental Health Go Hand in Hand

- Sleep detoxifies the brain, consolidates memory, and regulates emotions.
- Poor sleep increases stress hormones, lowers resilience, and worsens brain fog.
- A consistent sleep routine improves mood, focus, and overall well-being.
- Try This: Set a regular sleep schedule, reduce screen time before bed, and include magnesium-rich foods to improve sleep quality.

6.13 Take Action: Small Steps Lead to Lasting Change

- Start small. Choose one new habit to implement this week – adding gut-friendly foods, moving more, or prioritizing rest.
- Be patient. Mental health is a journey; every positive change builds toward long-term well-being.
- Stay consistent. Small, sustainable actions make the most significant impact overtime.

Your brain is adaptable. Your body is resilient. Your mental health is in your hands.

Final Thoughts: Inês's Advice for Whole-Body Healing

Inês reminds us that healing the mind starts with caring for the body. "I've seen time and again," she says, "how small, consistent habits – like eating better, sleeping well, or simply walking in nature – can transform mental health in ways medication alone can't." Her advice is simple: don't wait for crisis to act. Build daily habits that nourish both your emotional and physical self. Mental health is not a luxury – it's a foundation. And the best time to take that first step? Right now.

Your Healing Reflection:

- How closely do you feel your mental health and physical health are connected?
- What self-care practices could help support your emotional and physical well-being together?

Please complete the 'I will ...' statement on page 5.

Chapter Seven

Holistic Health & Behavior Change

Empowering Lasting Transformation Through Mindful Living

Ike, an immunologist, explains that chronic stress doesn't just drain your energy – it weakens your immune system, fuelling inflammation and leaving you vulnerable to illness.

Life is a whirlwind, isn't it? Stress can feel like an unwelcome companion when juggling work demands, family responsibilities, and personal aspirations. Imagine a typical day: a looming work deadline, the kids' extracurricular activities, and the endless cycle of meals and chores. Amidst this chaos, stress becomes an almost invisible thread, weaving through your life and impacting your health profoundly.

It's not just the mental strain; it's a physiological process that can create a cascade of inflammatory responses in your body. Understanding this connection between stress and inflammation is crucial, as it can empower you to make informed choices that promote well-being.

7.1 Stress and Inflammation: Understanding the Connection

When stress enters the scene, your body's response is both immediate and complex. It activates the hypothalamic-pituitary-adrenal (HPA) axis, a critical player in stress regulation. This system releases cortisol, a hormone designed to help you cope with stress.

- Short-term cortisol benefits: In short bursts, cortisol is beneficial, providing energy and focus.
- Chronic stress and cortisol levels: However, chronic stress keeps the HPA axis in overdrive, leading to persistently elevated cortisol levels. This dysregulation can wreak havoc on your body, exacerbating inflammation and contributing to a host of health issues, such as:
- Immune dysfunction
- Cardiovascular diseases

The constant release of cortisol under chronic stress conditions primes your immune system to remain in a heightened state, perpetuating inflammation and disrupting overall health balance.

7.2 The Impact of Stressors in Everyday Life

Stressors in everyday life are numerous, and their impact on health is significant. High-pressure jobs are a common source, particularly in today's fast-paced work environment. The relentless pursuit of deadlines and targets can leave you feeling overwhelmed, a sensation that lingers long after the workday ends. This stress doesn't just vanish; it accumulates, feeding into the cycle of inflammation.

- Emotional stressors: Emotional stressors, such as family dynamics, personal relationships, and financial worries, also play a substantial role. These stressors can be insidious, subtly influencing your mood and health over time. You might not always recognize the connection between an argument with a loved one or a looming bill and your body's inflammatory response, but it's there, quietly influencing your well-being.

7.3 Stress Management Techniques: Practical Solutions

To mitigate the effects of stress, adopting effective stress management techniques is essential. Progressive Muscle Relaxation (PMR) is a practical method for reducing tension. It involves systematically tensing and then relaxing different muscle groups, promoting physical relaxation and mental calm.

- The benefits of PMR: This technique can be particularly beneficial at the end of a long day, helping to release the accumulated stress that has settled in your muscles.

- Time management strategies: Time management skills are another valuable tool. By prioritizing tasks and setting realistic goals, you can reduce the overwhelming feeling that often accompanies a packed schedule. Breaking tasks into manageable chunks and setting clear boundaries between work and personal time can foster a sense of control and reduce stress levels.

7.4 Integrating Stress-Reduction Practices into Daily Life

Integrating stress-reduction practices into daily life is not just beneficial; it's necessary. Setting boundaries is a powerful strategy for limiting work-related stress. Consider designating specific times when work-related emails or tasks are off-limits, allowing you to fully engage with family or personal activities without distraction.

- Regular self-check-ins: Regular self-check-ins are equally important. These are moments when you pause to assess your current stress levels and emotional state. Ask yourself:
  - How am I feeling right now?
  - What is contributing to my stress?

This mindfulness, this reflection, helps you identify stressors early and address them before they escalate. Such practices encourage a proactive approach to stress management, ensuring that you maintain balance amidst life's demands.

7.5 Interactive Element: Stress Reflection Exercise

Take a few minutes each day to journal about your stress. Reflect on the following prompts:
- What triggered your stress today?
- How did your body respond to it (e.g., tension, fatigue)?
- What steps did you take to address or alleviate it?
- What could you do differently next time to manage stress more effectively?

Use this exercise to gain insights into your stress patterns and develop personalized strategies to reduce their impact on your health.

7.6 Cultivating Change: Strategies for Sustainable Habit Formation

Everyday life is filled with routines, from that first cup of coffee in the morning to the way you settle down to sleep each night. These routines, at their core, are habits – behaviors that have become automatic over time. Understanding how these habits form is the first step in changing them.

- The psychology behind habit formation: The psychology behind habit formation is fascinating yet simple. It revolves around a three-step loop: cue, routine, and reward.
- The cue is a trigger that prompts the habit, whether it's the time of day, a specific location, or a particular emotion.
- The routine is the behavior or action you perform.
- The reward reinforces the habit by providing a sense of satisfaction or relief.

This cycle strengthens neural pathways in your brain, making the behavior more automatic with each repetition.

7.7 Mindfulness Practices: Reducing Stress for Better Health

In the hustle and bustle of everyday life, we often yearn for a moment of peace – a moment to breathe, to be present. This is where mindfulness steps in, inviting you to focus on the here and now, enhancing awareness and reducing stress.

What is Mindfulness?

Mindfulness is the practice of focusing on the present moment without judgment.

- Focus on the present: Imagine starting your day with a few minutes of mindfulness, as you sit quietly, tuning into your breath and the sensations of the world around you. This practice shifts your attention away from the chaos, anchoring you in the present.
- Mindfulness in action: It is about observing your thoughts and feelings without judgment. When your mind wanders to worries or tasks, gently bring it back to the moment, accepting whatever arises with kindness. This non-judgmental observation fosters a sense of peace, reducing the mental clutter that can exacerbate stress.

Mindful Breathing & Body Scan Meditation

Mindfulness offers various techniques to integrate into daily routines, each designed to calm the mind and enhance awareness. One such technique is mindful breathing.

- Mindful breathing exercises: These involve focusing intently on your breath, noticing the rise and fall of your chest, the cool air entering your nostrils, and the warm air leaving. This focus on breath serves as a grounding force, calming the mind and reducing anxiety.
- Body scan meditation: This practice enhances awareness of physical sensations. As you lie or sit comfortably, guide your attention through each part of your body, noticing areas of tension or relaxation. It relaxes the body and heightens your connection to it, making you more attuned to its needs.

7.8 Mindful Eating: A Nourishing Experience

Mindful eating encourages you to savor each bite, noticing your food's flavors, textures, and aromas.

- Mindful eating benefits: This heightened awareness fosters a greater connection with your meals, transforming eating from a routine task into a nourishing experience.

7.9 Mindfulness and Stress-Related Inflammation

Mindfulness plays a crucial role in managing stress-induced inflammation by reducing stress hormones like cortisol. Chronic stress can lead to elevated cortisol levels, fuelling inflammation.

- Reducing cortisol with mindfulness: By promoting relaxation and present-moment awareness, mindfulness helps lower cortisol, mitigating its inflammatory effects. This reduction in stress hormones not only alleviates the physical symptoms of stress but also supports overall health, helping prevent chronic diseases linked to inflammation.

7.10 Everyday Mindfulness Practices: Making Time for Calm

Incorporating mindfulness into everyday activities can transform mundane tasks into moments of calm and reflection. Mindful commuting is one such practice, turning travel time into a meditative experience.

- Mindful commuting: Whether you're driving or taking public transport, focus on the sensations around you: the sound of the engine, the feel of the seat, and the sights passing by. Instead of rushing through the journey, allow yourself to be fully present, embracing the moment.

- Mindful listening: Another way to weave mindfulness into your day and enhance your relationships through attentive presence. When conversing with others, focus entirely on the speaker, noticing their words, tone, body language, and emotions. This deep listening fosters connection and empathy, enriching your interactions and reducing stress. Integrating mindfulness into these everyday moments creates a tapestry of awareness and calm that supports your health and well-being.

7.11 The Role of Sleep: Quality Rest as an Inflammatory Regulator

Sleep is often the first thing we sacrifice when life gets busy, yet its profound impact on health, particularly inflammation, cannot be overstated. Quality sleep is a natural regulator of inflammation, influencing how our bodies respond to stress and recover from daily wear and tear.

- Sleep and inflammation: When you sleep, your body enters a restorative state, reducing the production of inflammatory cytokines, proteins that can fuel inflammation if left unchecked. However, when sleep is disrupted, these cytokines increase, leading to heightened inflammatory responses.
- The importance of quality sleep: This connection highlights the importance of sleep in maintaining a balanced immune system. It's not just about getting enough hours of sleep, but ensuring those hours are restful and uninterrupted.

7.12 Disruptions to Circadian Rhythm: Impact on Immune Function

Disruptions to your circadian rhythm, the internal clock that governs sleep-wake cycles, can have a cascading effect on immune function. This rhythm is crucial for regulating various bodily processes, including the timing of hormone release, metabolism, and even cell repair.

- Circadian rhythm imbalance: When your circadian rhythm is out of sync – perhaps due to irregular sleep patterns, shift work, or excessive exposure to artificial light – the body's immune response can become impaired. This disruption can lead to an increase in inflammatory markers, making you more susceptible to illness and chronic conditions.

7.13 Sleep Disorders and Their Impact on Inflammation

Common sleep disorders like insomnia and sleep apnea further compound these issues. Insomnia, characterized by difficulty falling or staying asleep, leaves you feeling unrested and fatigued, which can exacerbate stress and inflammation.

- The risks of sleep apnea: Sleep apnea, a condition where breathing repeatedly stops and starts during sleep, is particularly concerning as it reduces oxygen flow, leading to increased blood pressure and inflammation. Both conditions contribute to a cycle of inadequate rest and heightened inflammation, which can worsen chronic health problems such as cardiovascular disease and metabolic disorders.

7.14 Improving Sleep Hygiene for Better Health

Improving sleep hygiene is a practical way to enhance sleep quality and duration. Start by creating a sleep-conducive environment. This means ensuring your bedroom is cool, dark, and quiet. Consider blackout curtains to block out light and a fan or white noise machine to drown out disturbances.

- Sleep hygiene tips: A comfortable mattress and pillows also play a key role in ensuring restful sleep. Establishing a consistent bedtime routine is equally important. Try to go to bed and wake up at the same time each day, even on weekends, to reinforce your body's natural sleep-wake cycle.
- Relaxation techniques: Incorporate relaxation techniques, like reading or taking a warm bath, to signal to your body that it's time to wind down. Never go to bed angry.

7.15 Prioritizing Sleep for Overall Health

Prioritizing sleep as a component of overall health is vital. In our fast-paced world, it's easy to view sleep as expendable, something to be sacrificed for more waking hours. Yet, quality rest is foundational to managing inflammation and supporting well-being.

- Viewing sleep as self-care: It's about finding a balance between sleep and lifestyle demands. View sleep as self-care, a non-negotiable part of your routine that allows you to recharge and perform at your best. By integrating rest into your busy schedule, you acknowledge the significant role it plays in health, much like nutritious food and regular exercise.

Embrace Sleep as Part of Your Health Regimen

Embrace sleep not as an indulgence, but as an essential part of your health regimen.

7.16 Closing Thoughts on Holistic Health & Behaviour Change

As we've explored, the path to better health is shaped by a holistic approach – one that nurtures the body, mind, and spirit. Ike, an immunologist, reminds us that long-term health isn't just about diet and exercise but also about managing inflammation through stress reduction and immune resilience. By embracing mindfulness, managing stress, and prioritising restorative sleep, we can create lasting habits that reduce inflammation and enhance our overall well-being.

The journey towards healthier living is not about perfection but progress – taking each step with intention, patience, and the understanding that every small change can lead to transformative results. Your immune system, much like your habits, thrives on consistency and balance. Remember, the power to cultivate lasting change lies within you.

Your Healing Reflection:

- What small, sustainable behaviour change feels most important for your health journey right now?
- What inner belief or mindset shift might help you succeed?

Please complete the 'I will ...' statement on page 5.

The Complete Auto-immune Guide
Combat Chronic Inflammation with Reliable Diet and Lifestyle Strategies to Transform Your Health and Feel Your Best

"The best way to find yourself is to lose yourself in the service of others." – Mahatma Gandhi

Can You Help Others by Sharing Your Journey?

Hi friend,

You've made it this far, and that means you're already on the path to better health. You've learned how inflammation works, what fuels it, and how small changes in your food and daily habits can make a big difference. Now, I'd love to ask you for a small favour that could help others just like you.

If you've found this book helpful – if a page made you feel hopeful, a tip helped you eat better, or a story made you feel seen – please take a minute to leave a review. Your voice matters. When you share what helped you, you're lighting the way for someone else who may be feeling ill, confused, stuck, or overwhelmed. It doesn't need to be fancy. Just a few words about what stood out or how this book helped you would mean the world. If you're able to, a photo review would be wonderful – it helps others connect with your journey in a real and inspiring way.

Here's how your review makes a difference: 1. It helps others discover the book 2. It gives hope to those who need a fresh start 3. It supports our growing community of empowered readers.

Your review could be the reason someone takes the first step towards feeling better. Thank you for being part of this journey. Let's keep going together,

Hemant

Chapter Eight

Addressing Common Objections

Overcoming Barriers to Health and Wellness

Imagine this: You're sitting around the dinner table, and a lively debate unfolds about the benefits of an anti-inflammatory diet. Your partner argues that these diets are too restrictive, while your kids insist they're only for those with chronic illnesses. But what if the way we eat affects not just physical health but mental well-being too? Research shows that food plays a critical role in brain function, mood regulation, and stress resilience – making diet a fundamental part of mental health care.

At the head of the table, Grandpa listens quietly. Once a busy lawyer who worked late nights and lived on convenience meals, he now struggles with chronic health issues and the premature aging that years of stress and poor nutrition have accelerated and regular hospital visits. He shakes his head and says, 'I wish I had known this sooner.' His words serve as a reminder – what we eat today shapes not only how we feel now, but how we age and function in the years ahead.

8.1 Breaking the Myth: Anti-Inflammatory Diets Are Restrictive

☐ Variety of Choices: An anti-inflammatory diet is a culinary adventure, offering a diverse array of delicious foods. From vibrant salads to hearty grain bowls, there is a world of flavors and textures to explore, catering to all tastes and preferences.

☐ Emphasis on Whole Foods: The key to an anti-inflammatory diet lies in whole foods – fruits like berries and apples, vegetables like leafy greens and cruciferous veggies, nuts, and legumes – which provide satisfying, healthful meals.

8.2 Breaking the Myth: Anti-Inflammatory Diets Are Not Only for Chronic Illnesses

Another pervasive myth is that anti-inflammatory diets are only beneficial for individuals suffering from chronic illnesses. This misconception overlooks the preventative benefits of such a diet.

☐ Preventative Health Benefits: An anti-inflammatory diet can benefit everyone, regardless of their current health status. By reducing inflammation, you can proactively manage age-related health changes and reduce the risk of chronic conditions such as heart disease, diabetes, and cognitive decline.

☐ Scientific Backing: Research unequivocally supports the idea that a diet rich in anti-inflammatory foods enhances metabolic processes and improves overall health. This solid scientific foundation empowers you to take control of your well-being with confidence.

8.3 The Role of Misinformation in Perpetuating Myths

These myths persist mainly due to misinformation and sensationalized dietary advice. The media often presents diets as one-size-fits-all solutions, leading to misunderstandings about their applicability and benefits.

☐ Media's Role in Misinformation: Headlines often exaggerate the restrictions of certain diets or suggest that such diets are only necessary for certain groups, further promoting the idea that anti-inflammatory diets are not suitable for everyone. For instance, a headline might claim that a specific "superfood" can cure all ailments, leading to misunderstandings about the actual benefits of the food.

☐ Critical Thinking: To accurately assess the benefits of an anti-inflammatory diet, it's essential to question the sources of these claims and seek reliable, evidence-based information.

8.4 Critical Evaluation of Health Claims

To navigate this sea of misinformation, developing the skills to evaluate health claims critically is crucial.

☐ Evaluate the Source: Begin by assessing the credibility of the source. Look for information published in reputable journals or provided by qualified health professionals.

☐ Beware of Sensational Headlines: Sensational headlines that promise quick fixes are often misleading and lack scientific support. Instead, focus on peer-reviewed research with a transparent methodology.

8.5 Interactive Element: Myth-Busting Checklist

Use this comprehensive checklist to navigate the sea of dietary information, empowering you to make informed decisions about your health. This tool will help you confidently embrace and integrate an anti-inflammatory diet into your lifestyle.

☐ Evaluate the Source: Check the author's credentials and the publication's reputation.

☐ Look for Evidence: Ensure claims are supported by peer-reviewed research.

☐ Avoid Sensationalism: Be skeptical of headlines that promise quick fixes.

☐ Check for Bias: Consider whether the information is sponsored or has a commercial interest.

8.6 Mindfulness Practices: Reducing Stress for Better Health

In the hustle and bustle of everyday life, we often yearn for peace – a moment to breathe, to be present. This is where mindfulness steps in. Mindfulness is a practice that invites you to focus on the here and now, enhancing awareness and reducing stress. Imagine starting your day with a few minutes of mindfulness as you sit quietly, tuning into your breath and the sensations of the world around you.

Key Benefits of Mindfulness:
- Enhances awareness and reduces stress.
- Anchors you in the present moment, helping to clear mental clutter.
- Encourages non-judgmental observation of your thoughts and feelings.

This simple yet profound practice shifts your attention away from chaos, anchoring you in the present. It is about observing your thoughts and feelings without judgment. When your mind wanders to worries or tasks, gently bring it back to the moment, accepting whatever arises with kindness. This non-judgmental observation fosters a sense of peace, reducing the mental clutter that can exacerbate stress.

8.7 Mindful Breathing: A Powerful Stress-Relief Tool

Mindful breathing exercises are a cornerstone of mindfulness practice. Focusing intently on your breath can significantly calm the mind and reduce stress. Noticing the rise and fall of your chest, the cool air entering your nostrils, and the warm air leaving help center your thoughts and promote relaxation.

Key Mindful Breathing Practices:
- Focus on the breath: Notice how your chest rises and falls.
- Inhale slowly: Deep breaths help activate the parasympathetic nervous system, which calms the body.
- Exhale with awareness: Feel the release of tension with each breath.

This simple focus on breath serves as a grounding force, helping to bring calm and reduce anxiety.

8.8 Body Scan Meditation: Enhancing Awareness of Physical Sensations

Another powerful mindfulness technique is body scan meditation, which enhances your awareness of physical sensations. As you sit or lie comfortably, guide your attention through each part of your body, noticing areas of tension or relaxation.

Key Points in Body Scan Meditation:
- Start from the toes and slowly work upwards.

- Focus on the physical sensations in each body part.
- Release tension as you notice it, bringing calm to each area.

This practice relaxes the body and enhances your connection with it, helping you become more attuned to your body's needs.

8.9 Mindful Eating: Connecting to Food and Reducing Stress

Mindful eating is a practice that can transform your relationship with food. By eating slowly and with full awareness, you can savour each bite and appreciate the flavours, textures, and aromas of your meal.

How to Practice Mindful Eating:
- Take smaller bites and chew each bite thoroughly.
- Focus on the sensory experience of eating: taste, texture, smell.
- Avoid distractions like TV or smartphones, allowing yourself to fully enjoy your meal.

This practice encourages you to slow down and appreciate the nourishment provided by food, creating a greater connection to your meals and improving digestion.

8.10 Mindfulness and Stress-Induced Inflammation

Mindfulness plays a crucial role in managing stress-induced inflammation by reducing stress hormones like cortisol. Chronic stress can lead to elevated cortisol levels, which fuel inflammation. By promoting relaxation and present-moment awareness, mindfulness helps lower cortisol, mitigating its inflammatory effects.

Mindfulness and Cortisol Reduction:
- Regular mindfulness practice helps lower cortisol, a key stress hormone.
- Reducing cortisol through mindfulness decreases the inflammatory response in the body.
- This can lead to better physical and emotional health over time.

This reduction in stress hormones not only alleviates the physical symptoms of stress but also supports overall health, helping prevent chronic diseases linked to inflammation.

8.11 Incorporating Mindfulness into Everyday Activities

Integrating mindfulness into daily activities can transform mundane tasks into moments of calm and reflection. One example is mindful commuting, which turns travel time into a meditative experience. Whether you're driving or taking public transport, focus on the sensations around you – the sound of the engine, the feel of the seat, and the sights passing by.

Ways to Practice Mindfulness in Daily Life:
- Mindful commuting: Pay attention to the sounds and feelings around you while travelling.
- Mindful listening: Focus entirely on the speaker's words, tone, and body language during conversations.

Instead of rushing through the journey, allow yourself to be fully present, embracing the moment.

8.12 Mindful Listening: Enhancing Relationships and Reducing Stress

Mindful listening is another way to incorporate mindfulness into your day. When conversing with others, focus entirely on the speaker—not just their words but also their tone, body language, and emotions.

Key Benefits of Mindful Listening:
- Strengthens relationships by fostering empathy and connection.
- Reduces stress by focusing on the present moment and avoiding distractions.
- Improves communication and understanding.

This deep listening fosters connection and empathy, enriching your interactions and reducing stress.

8.13 The Role of Sleep in Mindfulness and Inflammation

Sleep plays an essential role in maintaining overall health and managing inflammation. Quality sleep reduces the production of inflammatory cytokines, proteins that can fuel inflammation if left unchecked. When sleep is disrupted, these cytokines increase, leading to heightened inflammatory responses.

Key Points on Sleep and Inflammation:
- Quality sleep reduces inflammation by controlling cytokine production.
- Poor sleep disrupts circadian rhythms and elevates inflammation.
- Mindfulness can support better sleep quality by helping you relax before bedtime.

This connection highlights the importance of restful sleep in maintaining a balanced immune system. It's not just about getting enough sleep; it's about ensuring those hours are restful and uninterrupted.

8.14 Improving Sleep Hygiene for Better Health

Improving sleep hygiene is a practical way to enhance sleep quality and duration. Start by creating a sleep-conducive environment. This means ensuring your bedroom is cool, dark, and quiet.

Tips for Better Sleep Hygiene:
- Keep your bedroom cool and dark for optimal sleep.
- Seta consistent sleep schedule, going to bed and waking up at the same time daily.
- Practice relaxation techniques before bed, such as reading or taking a warm bath.

By incorporating these simple practices into your routine, you can ensure better sleep quality and overall health.

8.15 Closing Thoughts: Embracing Mindfulness for a Healthier Life

As explored in this chapter, managing stress and reducing inflammation are essential for long-term health. Mindfulness practices – such as mindful breathing, body scans, and mindful eating – can play a vital role in calming the mind, lowering stress hormones, and preventing chronic diseases. When combined with good sleep hygiene, mindfulness can become a cornerstone of overall well-being, offering a natural way to enhance mental and physical health.

However, it's important to remember that mindfulness is a practice that takes time to develop. It's not about achieving instant results but about creating sustainable habits you can integrate into your daily life. Just like physical exercise, the more you practice mindfulness, the greater the benefits will be, both in the short term and over the years.

8.16 Actionable Takeaways:

☐ Start by incorporating just one mindfulness technique into your daily routine. The key is consistency, whether mindful breathing, mindful eating, or mindful walking.

☐ Focus on improving your sleep hygiene to enhance your body's ability to manage stress and inflammation. Aim for restful, uninterrupted sleep each night.

☐ Use mindfulness as a tool not only for relaxation but also for better focus, emotional regulation, and decision-making in your daily life.

8.17 Final Reflection Exercise:

At the head of the table, Grandpa listens quietly. Once a busy lawyer who worked late nights and lived on convenience meals, he now struggles with chronic health issues and the premature aging that years of stress and poor nutrition have accelerated. He sighs and says, 'You know, tastebuds are the real determinants of health. People eat what is tasty, not necessarily what is good for them. I spent years choosing convenience over nourishment, and now I'm paying the price. If I had trained my tastebuds to appreciate real, wholesome food instead of processed junk, maybe things would be different today.' His words serve as a reminder – what we eat today shapes not only how we feel now, but how we age and function in the years ahead. Would you be shaking your head and saying to your grandchildren, 'I wish I had known this sooner.'

Reflective Prompt:

- When you think about making lifestyle changes, what personal objections or doubts come up for you?
- How could you gently reframe these to empower action?

Please complete the 'I will ...' statement on page 5.

Chapter Nine

PRACTICAL SOLUTIONS FOR BUSY LIFESTYLES

Simple Strategies for Staying Healthy on the Go

A Doctor's Dilemma: Finding Time for Health

Radha is a dedicated doctor who has spent years prioritizing her patients' well-being over hers. Long shifts, unpredictable hours, and hospital cafeteria meals have become her norm. But now, she faces a harsh reality – she has developed type 2 diabetes and gained significant weight. Her parents also live with diabetes, making her situation feel even more inevitable. But is it? What can she do, given her demanding schedule?

Knowing about the disease and prescribing medications isn't enough. Proper health comes from daily choices – eating, moving, and managing stress. The challenge isn't just knowledge; it's finding practical ways to implement healthy habits in a fast-paced life.

One of the most straightforward and effective strategies is meal prepping. Home cooking and bringing prepared meals to work are crucial steps in regaining control over health. Preparing meals at home ensures that ingredients are fresh, portions are balanced, and unnecessary additives are avoided. By bringing homemade meals to work, Radha can sidestep unhealthy cafeteria options and processed convenience foods, making it easier to stick to an anti-inflammatory diet. By dedicating a small window of time each week to preparing meals, Radha can ensure she has nutrient-dense, anti-inflammatory options ready to go, reducing the temptation of processed or high-sugar foods. Small, consistent actions can create a foundation for long-term health, even in the busiest lifestyles.

9.1 Introduction

In this chapter, we'll explore how minor adjustments – smart meal planning, efficient exercise strategies, and stress management techniques – can help busy professionals like Radha take control of their health without sacrificing their careers or personal lives.

9.2 How Meal Prepping Works

- Saves Time: By preparing meals in advance, you can free up time in your week to focus on other priorities.
- Reduces Stress: Knowing that healthy, anti-inflammatory meals are already prepped reduces the anxiety of last-minute cooking.
- Promotes Healthy Eating: Meals ready to go make it easier to stick to a balanced, anti-inflammatory diet.

This approach streamlines your week; it transforms your relationship with food, making it a source of empowerment rather than a rushed last-minute scramble.

The Concept of Meal Prepping

The concept of meal prepping is simple, yet its impact can be profound. At its core, meal prepping involves preparing large quantities of staples, such as grains and proteins, ahead of time. Imagine cooking a big batch of quinoa or brown rice, versatile grains that can serve as the foundation for numerous dishes.

How to Make It Work

- Staples: Focus on versatile grains and proteins.
- Variety: Pair grains with proteins like grilled chicken or roasted chickpeas. These combinations can be easily mixed and matched to create diverse meals throughout the week.
- Timesaving: By investing a few hours upfront, you can free yourself from the daily grind of meal prep, giving you time to focus on other priorities.

Meal prepping allows you to maintain your health commitment without the stress of last-minute preparation.

9.3 Efficient Storage Solutions

Efficient storage solutions are key to successful meal prepping. Investing in quality containers can make a huge difference in keeping your meals fresh and organized.

Storage Tips

- Airtight containers: Look for containers that are stackable, airtight, and easy to clean.
- Glass containers: These are popular because they're durable, don't retain odors, and let you easily see what's inside.
- Mason jars: Perfect for salads or parfaits, mason jars are a great option for meals on the go. Layer ingredients strategically to create grab-and-go meals that stay fresh and delicious.
  - Metal containers: Excellent for freezing, as they're free from microplastics, highly durable, and non-porous. Stainless steel is a good choice for those avoiding plastic entirely.
  - Avoid plastic where possible: Repeated use and heating of plastic containers can release microplastics and endocrine-disrupting chemicals. Opt for glass or metal to protect both your health and the environment.

Choosing safer materials not only preserves the integrity of your meals - it can also reduce toxic exposure and inspire creativity as you explore vibrant, nourishing recipes.

This method not only helps preserve the integrity of your meals but also sparks creativity as you experiment with different flavor combinations.

9.4 Quick Anti-Inflammatory Recipes

When it comes to quick anti-inflammatory recipes, variety is the spice of life.

Simple Recipe Ideas

- Mason jar salads: Layer greens, quinoa, beans, and a rainbow of vegetables, then top with a zesty dressing. These salads are visually appealing and packed with nutrients, providing a satisfying, health-boosting meal in minutes.

☐ One-pan roasted vegetables: Toss seasonal produce with olive oil, spices, garlic, and rosemary. Roast to perfection for a medley of flavors and textures. These veggies can be enjoyed alone or paired with grains and proteins.

These recipes are designed to cater to diverse tastes and dietary needs, ensuring there's something for everyone.

9.5 Must-Have Gadgets

Certain tools and equipment can make meal prepping more efficient and enjoyable.

Kitchen Gadgets for Meal Prepping

☐ Slow cookers and Instant Pots are perfect for "set-it-and-forget-it" cooking. Imagine coming home to a comforting stew, ready to nourish you after a busy day.

☐ Blenders: Great for mornings on the go. A handful of spinach, a banana, and some flaxseeds can create a nutrient-dense smoothie that energizes your day.

These gadgets simplify the cooking process, making it easier to maintain healthy habits even when time is scarce.

9.6 Keeping Things Fresh Variety is key to keep your meals exciting and avoid the dreaded meal prep fatigue.

How to Keep Things Fresh

☐ Rotating ingredients weekly: This helps breathe new life into your meals, keeping your taste buds engaged.

☐ Seasonal produce: Explore the bounty of each season – spring brings the sweetness of asparagus and peas, while autumn offers the earthy flavors of squash and root vegetables.

☐ Flavored infusions: Infuse olive oil with chili flakes or lemon zest for a zesty kick. Steep herbs like basil or mint in vinegar for a refreshing dressing.

These small changes can elevate a simple dish into something truly special, and meal prepping allows you to get creative in the kitchen.

9.7 Interactive Element: Meal Prep Planner

Here's a simple plan to organize your week:

- ☐ Staples: Choose one grain and one protein to batch cook.
- ☐ Recipes: Select three recipes to prep (e.g., mason jar salads or roasted veggies).
- ☐ Tools: List the gadgets you'll use (e.g., slow cooker or blender).
- ☐ Flavors: Choose two infusions or spice blends to experiment with.
- ☐ Shopping List: Write down the ingredients needed for the week.

Keep this planner on your fridge as a reminder of your meal prep goals, ensuring each week is filled with delicious and healthful meals.

9.8 Technology in Meal Planning

Technology has become essential in managing our health in today's digital age. Imagine having a personal assistant in your pocket, always ready to organize your grocery lists and help plan your meals.

How Technology Can Help

- ☐ Meal planning apps: Apps like Mealime and PlateJoy allow you to digitally assemble recipes, plan weekly menus, and easily create grocery lists. These tools make meal planning easy and fun, offering customizable meal plans to cater to various dietary needs and preferences.
- ☐ Tailored suggestions: These apps provide nutritional data and suggestions that align with your health goals, helping you stay on track with your anti-inflammatory eating plan.
- ☐ Streamlining your shopping: These apps can simplify grocery shopping and ensure your pantry is stocked with anti-inflammatory ingredients, reducing the temptation to opt for less healthy options.

By embracing technology, you can make healthy eating more manageable and efficient.

9.9 Fitness Trackers Supporting Your Wellness

Beyond meal planning, fitness trackers have revolutionized how we monitor physical activity.

How Fitness Trackers Can Support Your Wellness

- ☐ Beyond step counting: These devices offer insights into your overall activity levels, heartrate, and even sleep patterns. Think of them as a personal coach, always thereto encourage you to move more and achieve your fitness targets.

- Comprehensive tracking: Devices like Fitbit and Garmin not only track your activities but also sync with other health apps, creating a comprehensive picture of your wellness journey.
- Motivation through feedback: By setting daily goals and receiving real-time feedback, fitness trackers help keep you motivated to stay active, even during busy times. The accountability these devices offer can be a powerful motivator, pushing you to prioritize physical activity in your daily routine.

With fitness trackers, staying on top of your physical health becomes more manageable and motivating.

9.10 Enhancing Mental Well-being with Technology

In addition to supporting physical health, technology can also enhance your mental well-being.

How Technology Supports Mental Health
- Meditation apps: Apps like Headspace and Calm offer guided sessions that help you relax and focus, providing a moment of calm amidst your busy day.
- Variety of options: Whether you're looking to reduce stress, improve sleep, or increase mindfulness, these apps cater to various needs. Choose from quick, three-minute breathing exercises or more in-depth meditation sessions that fit your lifestyle.
- Breathing exercises: Many apps integrate breathing exercises, teaching techniques that lower stress levels and improve mental clarity.

Using these tools, you can incorporate mindfulness into your daily routine, fostering peace and balance.

9.11 Choosing the Right Tech Tools

Selecting the right tech tools requires careful consideration.

How to Choose the Right Tools
- User reviews and ratings: Start by checking reviews and ratings. Positive feedback often indicates reliability and satisfaction, offering insights into an app's effectiveness and user-friendliness.

- Customizable features: Look for apps with personalization features. Whether adjusting notifications or choosing content types, customization ensures the app aligns with your unique goals.
- Free trials: Use free trials to explore the app's capabilities before committing to a purchase. This allows you to test the app's functionality and assess how well it integrates into your daily routine.

Choosing the right app can empower you to manage your health more effectively, making it easier to stick to your wellness goals.

9.12 Balancing Tech Use

While technology offers numerous benefits, it's important to be mindful of its potential drawbacks.

Strategies for Balancing Tech Use

- Screen time management: Set boundaries for device usage, especially before bedtime. This ensures that technology enhances your life without taking over.
- "Tech-free" zones: Consider creating tech-free spaces or times in your home to encourage face-to-face interactions and reduce screen fatigue.
- Privacy concerns: When choosing apps, always review their data protection policies to understand how your information is used and stored. Opt for apps that prioritize user privacy, offering transparent and secure data practices.

By taking these precautions, you can harness technology's power while protecting your well-being.

Conclusion:

A year later, Radha reflects on her journey and the difference small, consistent changes have made. 'I used to believe I had no time for healthy eating or exercise, but I've learned that prioritizing my health doesn't mean overhauling my entire life – it just means being intentional with my choices. Meal prepping became my lifeline. Instead of relying on cafeteria food, I now bring homemade meals to work, and it has transformed my energy levels and blood sugar control. I also found ways to incorporate movement into my day, even during hospital shifts – taking the stairs, stretching between patients, and making time for short walks.'

Radha's experience proves that even in the busiest of lives, small steps create meaningful change. By focusing on manageable adjustments rather than drastic transformations, she reversed unhealthy patterns and built habits that support her long-term well-being. Radha's journey is a reminder that even the busiest professionals can reclaim their health with small, intentional changes. Knowing about disease is not enough – real transformation comes from consistent, daily actions. By embracing meal prepping, home cooking, and simple lifestyle adjustments, she can break free from the cycle of poor eating habits and take control of her well-being.

Your Healing Reflection:

- What are the biggest obstacles you face when trying to live healthily day-to-day?

- Which practical solutions from this chapter would fit most naturally into your life?

Please complete the 'I will ...' statement on page 5.

CHAPTER TEN

EXPLORING THE WORLD THROUGH FOOD – A CULINARY JOURNEY

HEALING THROUGH GLOBAL FLAVORS AND NOURISHMENT

A New Way of Eating: Grandma Gertrude's Story

For most of her life, Grandma Gertrude's diet consisted of classic American staples – burgers, fried foods, and sugary treats. She never considered venturing beyond the familiar until a wake-up call forced her to rethink everything. After years of routine eating, she found herself overweight, struggling with high blood pressure, and facing serious health concerns.

That's when her Chinese nutritionist introduced her to a world of vibrant, diverse, and nourishing foods. By embracing a more varied diet filled with colorful vegetables, fiber-rich grains, and healing spices, Gertrude saw remarkable changes. She shed excess weight, regained her energy, and discovered a new passion for food. Today, she's not just healthier – she's thriving. She runs half marathons, experiments with global cuisines, and even hosts dinner parties featuring dishes inspired by cultures around the world.

Gertrude's story is proof that food is more than just sustenance – it's an adventure, a pathway to better health, and a way to connect with others. In this chapter, we'll explore how expanding your culinary horizons can nourish your body, improve your health, and enrich your life.

10.1 Introduction

Imagine yourself in your kitchen, surrounded by various ingredients from around the world. The vibrant colors of fresh produce, aromatic spices, and fragrant herbs create a sensory experience that excites you as you prepare for a culinary journey. These ingredients offer more than just nourishment – they transport you to different lands, each with its own culture, history, and traditions. Cooking becomes a celebration of global flavors, an exploration of diverse cuisines, and a powerful way to enhance your health. And when you share these meals, you're not just eating; you're building a community, connecting with others through a shared love of food.

By integrating cultural influences into your diet, you're embracing the richness of global cuisines and reaping the health benefits that come with them. Each culture brings unique, health-boosting ingredients and cooking methods that support your well-being. From anti-inflammatory spices to nutrient-dense vegetables, this journey through food is both a cultural exploration and a path to better health, helping you feel more energized and nourished.

10.2 How Cultural Diets Enhance Health

Incorporating diverse dietary practices into your meals can profoundly impact your health, offering a variety that balances your palate and nutrient intake. Here's how different cultural cuisines contribute to overall wellness:

Mediterranean Diet

The Mediterranean diet is more than just a collection of recipes; it's a lifestyle rich in healthy fats, antioxidants, and whole foods.

- Healthy Fats: Emphasizes plant-based foods such as whole grains, olive oil, and nuts.
- Omega-3 Fatty Acids: Fish, particularly rich in omega-3s, is a staple, supporting heart health.

- Moderate Red Meat Consumption: Focuses on plant-based foods and seafood, with limited red meat intake.

Health Benefits of the Mediterranean Diet

By adopting elements of this diet, you can reduce your risk of heart disease while enjoying flavorful and nourishing meals. Its emphasis on antioxidants and omega-3 fatty acids also supports brain function and longevity.

Japanese Cuisine: A Path to Longevity

Japanese cuisine offers another perspective on healthy eating, renowned for its contribution to longevity.

- Emphasis on Fresh, Seasonal Ingredients: Staples include fish, vegetables, and rice, with minimal processed foods.
- Fermented Foods: Incorporates miso and natto, which support gut health and digestion.
- Nutrient-Dense & Low-Calorie: Seaweed, rich in iodine and other minerals, promotes thyroid health and overall well-being.

By focusing on fresh, nutrient-dense ingredients, Japanese cuisine enhances flavor and supports long-term health and longevity.

10.3 Culinary Exploration & Expanding Your Palate

Variety is not just the spice of life – it's essential in preventing dietary monotony and ensuring adherence to healthy eating habits. Incorporating diverse cuisines into your weekly meals enhances both your health and culinary experience.

- Prevents Boredom & Encourages Healthier Choices: Rotating different cultural cuisines in meal planning avoids monotony and reduces reliance on processed foods.

- Promotes Balanced Nutrient Intake: A diverse range of dishes provides essential antioxidants, healthy fats, and fiber.

- Enhances Culinary Engagement: Exploring different cuisines turns healthy eating into an adventure rather than a chore.

- Supports Social and Cultural Connection: Sharing meals inspired by global traditions fosters a deeper appreciation of food cultures and strengthens bonds through communal eating.

10.4 Exploring Global Cuisines

Certain cultural cuisines are known for their health-promoting properties. One example is the Nordic diet, which emphasizes whole grains, fish, and root vegetables while aligning closely with sustainability principles.

- Rich in Fiber & Healthy Fats: Root vegetables provide fiber, while salmon and other fatty fish offer heart-healthy omega-3s.
- Supports Cardiovascular & Brain Health: Omega-3s reduce inflammation and promote cognitive function.
- Encourages Sustainable Eating: Focuses on seasonal, locally sourced ingredients for environmental and health benefits.

Curiosity and exploration in culinary practices open the door to endless possibilities, encouraging you to venture beyond familiar flavors. Engaging in food festivals and cooking classes provides immersive opportunities to learn about and taste different cuisines.

- Expanding Your Culinary Repertoire: Food festivals introduce authentic dishes, deepening appreciation for global flavors.
- Learning New Techniques: Hands-on cooking classes provide expert guidance on traditional preparation methods.
- Enhancing Creativity: Experimenting with new ingredients and techniques keeps meals exciting and nutrient-rich.

10.5 Interactive Element: Culinary Exploration Checklist

Exploring diverse cultural influences through your cooking journey can be rewarding. Use this checklist to guide your culinary adventure:

- Attend a Local Food Festival – Immerse yourself in authentic flavors and learn about different cuisines' cultural significance.
- Enroll in a Cooking Class – Learn techniques from expert chefs specializing in global cuisines.
- Try a New Cuisine Weekly – Challenge yourself to incorporate international flavors into your meal planning for variety and excitement.
- Visit Ethnic Markets – Source authentic ingredients and spices to add authenticity to your meals.

- ☐ Start a Food Diary – Document your culinary experiences, noting favorite recipes and new techniques.

10.6 Respectful Integration: Adopting Ethnic Practices Mindfully

As you explore global flavors, it's crucial to approach each cuisine with respect and understanding. Every dish carries a story – a reflection of traditions, values, and cultural heritage. By embracing the roots of these dishes, you deepen your appreciation for diverse culinary traditions.

Engage with Cultural Experts and Authentic Sources

To adopt ethnic culinary practices in a meaningful way:

- ☐ Learn from Trusted Sources – Read books, watch documentaries, and follow chefs who specialize in traditional cuisine.
- ☐ Understand the Significance of Ingredients – Research the cultural background behind key ingredients and their role in traditional dishes.
- ☐ Follow Traditional Techniques – When making sushi, for example, practice authentic rice preparation and rolling methods to preserve its true essence.

Preserving Original Cooking Techniques

When recreating traditional recipes, strive to maintain authenticity:

- ☐ Respect the Culinary Heritage – Honor the cultural origins of dishes by following traditional preparation methods.
- ☐ Maintain Authenticity – Using original cooking methods ensures dishes retain their intended flavors and textures.
- ☐ Explore the Process – Mastering traditional techniques enhances your culinary skills while preserving cultural integrity.

10.7 Healthy Global Recipes & Anti-Inflammatory Ingredients

Many global dishes incorporate ingredients known for their anti-inflammatory properties. For instance:

Indian Lentil Dal

A staple in Indian cuisine, dal is rich in protein, fiber, and anti-inflammatory spices.

- ☐ Turmeric & Cumin: Contain powerful antioxidants that combat inflammation.
- ☐ Lentils: Provide plant-based protein and support digestive health.

- Lemon: Adds a vitamin C boost, enhancing nutrient absorption and immunity.

Vietnamese Pho

A fragrant noodle soup packed with nutrient-dense ingredients.

- Bone Broth: Supports gut health and provides essential minerals.
- Star Anise & Cloves: Contain compounds that support immune function.
- Fresh Herbs: Cilantro and basil add flavor and antioxidants.

By exploring and respecting the origins of anti-inflammatory recipes from around the world, you can enrich your meals while deepening your connection to global culinary traditions. At the same time, incorporating diverse, nutrient-rich ingredients ensures your body receives essential vitamins, minerals, and antioxidants that help combat inflammation. From the turmeric in Indian curries, known for its powerful curcumin content, to the omega-3 fatty acids in Mediterranean cuisine that support heart health, embracing these traditional dishes not only enhances flavour but also nurtures overall well-being.

10.8 Building Community Through Food

Food is not just sustenance – it's a powerful tool for connection. Sharing meals strengthens relationships and fosters a sense of unity.

- Family Dinners: Encourage communication and reinforce traditions.
- Community Gatherings: Hosting international potlucks allows for cultural exchange.
- Cultural Storytelling: Learning the origins of dishes adds depth to the dining experience.

10.9 Reflections & Actionable Steps

By embracing the richness of global cuisines, you nourish both your body and mind. Here are some steps to take your culinary journey further:

- Attend Local Food Festivals: Immerse yourself in authentic flavors and traditions.
- Experiment with New Recipes Weekly: Keep meals exciting and nutrient-dense.
- Source Authentic Ingredients: Visit ethnic markets for genuine flavors.
- Respect Culinary Traditions: Learn from cultural experts and preserve original techniques.

By exploring food through a global lens, you cultivate appreciation for diverse traditions while enriching your health and well-being. Enjoy the journey, one meal at a time!

10.10 The Role of Ingredients in Health Benefits

The ingredients and techniques unique to different global recipes play a crucial role in their health benefits. Some key components include:

- Fresh Herbs and Spices – Enhance both flavor and nutrition while offering anti-inflammatory and antioxidant properties.
- Fermented Foods – Such as kimchi and miso, introduce beneficial probiotics that support gut health.
- Probiotics – Aid digestion and improve nutrient absorption, contributing to overall wellness.

By embracing these techniques, you enrich your meals and support your body's natural functions, making each meal a step toward better health.

10.11 Encouraging Experimentation with Global Recipes

Bringing diversity into the kitchen by experimenting with global recipes makes cooking more exciting and engaging. Consider these practices:

- International Night: Dedicate one night a week to exploring a new international cuisine. It can be a fun family event where everyone participates in selecting or preparing the meal.
- Recipe Variety: Try a Moroccan tagine one week and a Thai green curry the next. This keeps your meals interesting and introduces your family to new flavors and traditions.

By diversifying your meals, you transform dinner into an adventure rather than a routine.

10.12 Finding Authentic Ingredients

Finding authentic ingredients is part of the joy of cooking global dishes. Consider these tips:

- Local Ethnic Markets: These markets offer spices, sauces, and fresh produce that can transform your cooking, providing access to hard-to-find items that add authenticity to your meals.
- Online Specialty Shops: If local markets do not carry what you need, specialty online stores provide a convenient alternative, ensuring you access authentic international ingredients.

By sourcing authentic components, you ensure your dishes remain true to their origins, respecting the culinary traditions they represent.

10.13 Global Cuisine as a Journey

The world of global cuisine offers an endless array of possibilities, with each dish serving as a testament to the creativity and resourcefulness of its culture. As you explore these recipes, here's what you'll find:

- Connection to Culture: Cooking global dishes becomes more than a daily task; it's a way to connect with the world. Each meal offers a journey through different traditions.
- Culinary Experimentation: Embrace the opportunity to try different cooking techniques and ingredients. This creativity enriches your culinary experience and supports your well-being.

Allow the flavors to inspire you, and enjoy the health benefits with every bite.

10.14 Sharing the Table: Building Community Through Diverse Meals

In every home, the dining table is more than just a place to eat; it is a space where connections deepen, and cultures come alive. Sharing a meal fosters a sense of belonging and unity. Here's how:

- Family Dinners: Sitting down together improves communication, reinforces traditions, and creates lasting memories.
- Community Gatherings: Hosting an international potluck allows everyone to share their heritage and build mutual respect.
- Celebrating Diversity: We celebrate the richness of various cultures and the stories behind each dish through food.

These shared experiences bring joy and remind us of food's power to unite.

10.15 Learning Through Culinary Traditions

Each dish carries more than just flavor and health benefits; it holds a story, a piece of history. By learning about the origins of these dishes, you:

- Appreciate the Heritage: Understanding the history behind a dish fosters respect for the traditions and values that created it.
- Strengthen Connections: Sharing the stories behind the food adds depth to the dining experience and creates bonds.
- Celebrate Generations of Wisdom: By embracing cultural practices, you honor the generations who have perfected these recipes.

This knowledge transforms eating into a health improving celebration of the cultures and histories we are privileged to experience.

10.16 The Power of Sharing Meals

Meals are not only an opportunity to nourish ourselves but also a chance to connect with others. Sharing food brings people together and strengthens community bonds. You can experience this by:

- Hosting a Potluck: Invite friends and neighbors to bring dishes from their heritage. This fosters cultural exchange and community spirit.
- Themed Dinners: Organize dinners where you explore the cuisine of a particular country, offering guests an opportunity to experience new tastes and traditions.
- Learning Through Stories: Each dish has a story. By sharing those stories, you gain deeper insight into the traditions that shaped the food.

Sharing meals this way builds empathy and respect while enriching your culinary knowledge.

10.17 Health Benefits of Cultural Diversity on the Table

Exploring different cultural foods enriches your culinary knowledge and offers significant health benefits. Each cuisine brings unique ingredients and techniques that support overall wellness:

- ☐ Incorporating Nutrient-Dense Ingredients: Many global diets include nutrient-dense foods like leafy greens, seeds, and legumes. These foods are rich in essential vitamins and minerals that support immune function, digestion, and heart health.
- ☐ Boosting Antioxidant Intake: Spices and herbs from various cuisines, such as turmeric, ginger, and cilantro, are known for their anti-inflammatory and antioxidant properties, helping reduce inflammation and improve overall health.
- ☐ Balanced Diets for Long-Term Health: By integrating cultural meals into your routine, you can create a balanced diet that includes a variety of nutrient-rich foods, promoting longevity, mental clarity, and a healthy weight.

Conclusion: A World of Health at Your Table

By embracing the wide variety of global cuisines, you'll enjoy exciting new flavors and nourish your body with a broader spectrum of health-enhancing ingredients. Different cultures have long understood the healing power of food – whether it's the anti-inflammatory spices of India, the gut-friendly fermented foods of Korea, or the heart-healthy Mediterranean diet. Expanding your culinary horizons means giving your body access to a rich diversity of nutrients, antioxidants, and beneficial compounds that support overall well-being.

Food is more than just sustenance – it's a gateway to better health, deeper connections, and a greater appreciation of the world around you. By stepping beyond familiar comfort foods and exploring new traditions, you can transform your meals into a powerful tool for longevity and vitality.

Your Healing Reflection:

- Which global cuisines are you most excited to explore to diversify your meals?
- How can you make culinary exploration a regular part of your healthy eating journey?

Please complete the 'I will ...' statement on page 5.

Chapter Eleven

Science-Backed Approaches to Healing and Wellness

Grounding Health Solutions in Research and Proven Results

A **Wake-Up Call: Ade's Journey into Food Awareness**

Before becoming a father, Ade rarely gave much thought to food labels. He grabbed whatever was convenient, trusting that if it was on the supermarket shelf, it was safe to eat. But everything changed when his newborn daughter developed severe food allergies. Suddenly, he found himself meticulously reading every ingredient list, scanning for hidden allergens, and questioning what was really in the foods he had been consuming for years.

As he dug deeper, he was shocked to discover the additives, preservatives, and artificial ingredients lurking in everyday products. He realised that food wasn't just about taste and convenience – it was about quality, safety, and long-term health. This new awareness led him to embrace evidence-based nutrition, making informed choices not only for his daughter but for himself and his entire family.

Ade's journey highlights the power of knowledge in transforming health. In this chapter, we'll explore how evidence-based practices – grounded in science and careful evaluation – can help you navigate misleading food labels, distinguish between marketing hype and real nutrition, and take control of your well-being with confidence.

Inspired by Ade's story, let us, once again, imagine starting your day with a warm cup of coffee, scrolling through the latest health news. With so much scientific research available, it's easy to feel overwhelmed. Studies filled with complex jargon and conflicting information can make it difficult to separate fact from fiction. But understanding research doesn't have to be intimidating. With the right approach, you can gain the skills to interpret scientific findings and make well-informed health decisions with confidence.

11.1 Types of Research Studies

Scientific studies come in different forms, each serving a specific purpose in advancing our understanding of health and disease.

Observational Studies

Researchers observe people in their everyday environments without interfering. These studies can identify connections between behaviors and health outcomes but cannot confirm direct cause-and-effect relationships.

Clinical Trials

These controlled studies actively test interventions, like new treatments or dietary changes, to evaluate their effects. Many clinical trials use randomization (where participants are assigned by chance) and blinding (where neither researchers nor participants know who receives the treatment) to ensure reliable results.

Meta-Analysis

These studies combine data from multiple smaller studies, analyzing results from a larger group of participants to provide a more comprehensive picture of a health trend.

11.2 Assessing Credibility

Not all research is created equal, so knowing how to evaluate a study's reliability is essential.

Peer review plays a critical role in ensuring the quality of published research. In this process, independent experts assess a study before it is accepted for publication, helping to filter out poorly conducted research. If a study is peer-reviewed, it has undergone this level of scrutiny, making it more trustworthy.

However, even peer-reviewed studies can have biases. Those interests may influence research funded by companies with financial interests in specific outcomes. Similarly, researchers may have personal or professional biases that shape their interpretations. Before trusting a study, check who funded it and whether any conflicts of interest could affect its conclusions.

11.3 Common Pitfalls in Interpreting Research

Understanding research requires recognizing some common mistakes people make when interpreting findings.

Correlation vs. Causation

Just because two things happen together doesn't mean one causes the other. For example, a study may show that people who eat more olive oil tend to have lower heart disease rates, but that doesn't prove olive oil is the reason for better heart health.

Overgeneralization

Study results apply to specific conditions and populations. A study conducted on young athletes may not be relevant to older adults. Always check whether the study population reflects your situation before applying its findings to your life.

11.4 Real-World Example: The Mediterranean Diet

Scientific research has repeatedly linked diet to inflammation. One example is the Mediterranean diet, which is rich in vegetables, fruits, olive oil, and fish.

A well-designed randomized controlled trial found that participants who followed the Mediterranean diet experienced significant reductions in joint pain and stiffness associated with rheumatoid arthritis. Another study focusing on omega-3 fatty acids – abundant in fatty fishlike salmon – demonstrated that these healthy fats help lower inflammation and improve arthritis symptoms.

11.5 Reflection Exercise: Evaluating Health Studies

Next time you come across a health study, take a moment to analyze it critically. Ask yourself:

- What type of study was it – observational, clinical trial, or meta-analysis?
- Was the sample size large enough to support the findings?
- Did the study include control groups to improve validity?
- Was the study peer-reviewed, and who funded it?
- Are the conclusions relevant to your health and lifestyle?

Developing the skill to assess research thoughtfully empowers you to make informed choices that align with your health goals. The more you question and evaluate studies, the more confident you'll apply evidence-based practices.

11.6 The Science of Spices: Validating Their Health Benefits

Picture yourself in the kitchen, surrounded by the enticing aromas of spices. These aren't just flavor enhancers; they are regarded as powerful health allies. Research is increasingly validating the medicinal properties of spices that have been used in traditional medicine for centuries.

Curcumin

Curcumin is recognized as an active compound in turmeric, known for its potent anti-inflammatory and antioxidant effects. It has been suggested by studies that conditions such as arthritis and metabolic syndrome can be managed with curcumin. However, the bio availability of curcumin, which refers to the amount absorbed and used by the body, is considered low. This means that even when a certain amount of curcumin is consumed, not all of it may be utilized by the body. To enhance absorption, curcumin is often combined with piperine, a compound found in black pepper, which has been shown to increase curcumin absorption by up to 2000%.

Cinnamon

This spice is not only used to add warmth to oatmeal but has also been shown to provide health benefits. The compound cinnamaldehyde in cinnamon has been linked to the regulation of blood sugar, which is considered crucial for managing diabetes and maintaining stable energy levels throughout the day. Research supports its role in the prevention of diabetes-related complications.

Garlic

The active compound in garlic, allicin, has been shown to lower LDL cholesterol (the "bad" cholesterol) and improve vascular health. Antimicrobial properties have also been attributed to garlic, and it is recognized for supporting immune function.

Ginger

Ginger is widely known for its effectiveness in easing nausea. It has been found to reduce nausea caused by pregnancy, chemotherapy, and surgery. Gingerol and shogaol have been identified as interacting with serotonin receptors in the gut to provide relief.

Spices can easily be incorporated into the daily diet. For example, a turmeric latte (prepared using turmeric, warm milk, and black pepper) can be consumed in the morning, or cinnamon can be sprinkled on oatmeal to enhance both flavor and health benefits.

11.7 Understanding the Challenges in Spice Research

Unlike synthetic compounds, spices are natural products, meaning their composition can vary. The potency of spices has been found to be affected by factors such as growing conditions and processing methods, making standardization of research difficult. Additionally, the influence of different cultural uses of spices on their perceived effectiveness has been acknowledged.

11.8 Nutrition Myths vs. Facts: Clarifying Common Misconceptions

With so much information available, misconceptions can easily spread. One of the most common is the belief that all fats are unhealthy. This misconception originated from the low-fat diet trend of past decades, which blamed fats for weight gain and heart disease. However, not all fats are the same. Healthy fats, such as omega-3 fatty acids found in fish, nuts, and seeds, have been found to be crucial for heart health and reducing inflammation.

Another widespread myth is that carbohydrates should be avoided. Complex carbohydrates, such as those in wholegrains and vegetables, have been recognized as essential for energy. They provide sustained energy and help regulate blood sugar levels. However, refined carbohydrates—such as white bread and sugary snacks—have been shown to cause rapid blood sugar spikes, which can lead to weight gain and inflammation.

11.9 Navigating Misinformation

Misinformation has been found to lead to poor health choices, including adherence to fad diets and extreme restrictions. These diets, while promising quick fixes, have been associated with nutrient deficiencies and long-term health risks. Instead of following short-term trends, the importance of balance and nutrition should be emphasized. By understanding the significance of a balanced diet, informed decisions can be made, reducing the likelihood of falling for misleading quick-fix solutions.

11.10 Trusted Resources: Where to Find Reliable Health Information

With the vast amount of health information available online, identifying trustworthy sources is crucial. The following are recognized as reliable sources:

1. Academic Journals: Peer-reviewed journals are widely regarded as the gold standard for reliable research.

2. Government Health Websites: Websites such as the National Institutes of Health (NIH) and the Centers for Disease Control and Prevention(CDC) provide up-to-date and trustworthy information.

3. Health Professionals: Registered dietitians and doctors are acknowledged as sources of personalized advice based on the latest research.

Relying on these trusted resources can help make well-informed health decisions, ensuring that choices are based on credible and scientifically supported information.

Conclusion: From Awareness to Advocacy

A year later, Ade's journey into food awareness transformed his family's health and his community. What began as a desperate search for safe foods for his daughter evolved into a passion for evidence-based nutrition. He became the go-to resource for other parents navigating food allergies and label confusion, sharing insights on avoiding hidden additives, understanding nutritional claims, and making healthier choices.

By prioritizing informed decisions, Ade ensured that his family thrived on whole, nutrient-rich foods while reducing reliance on overly processed options. Their diet became both anti-inflammatory and diverse, incorporating a wide range of whole grains, lean proteins, healthy fats, and colorful vegetables. Inspired by different global cuisines, Ade experimented with spices, fermented foods, and nutrient-dense ingredients that supported gut health and overall well-being. He discovered that true health isn't just about eliminating harmful ingredients – it's about embracing real, nourishing foods that fuel the body and mind.

His story is a testament to the power of knowledge. When we take the time to learn, question, and apply evidence-based practices, we gain more than just better health – we gain the confidence to make choices that positively impact those around us. Through small, intentional steps, anyone can transition from uncertainty to empowerment, creating a ripple effect of well-being in their families and communities.

Your Healing Reflection:

- How has understanding the science behind inflammation and healing shifted your motivation?

- Which evidence-based strategy do you feel most inspired to implement?

Please complete the 'I will ...' statement on page 5.

Chapter Twelve

Digital, Community and Global Engagement

Connecting People and Technology for Global Wellness

The Power of Collective Well-being

A healthy community doesn't merely exist - its members' participation and engagement actively shape it. Beyond having access to nutritious foods, safe spaces for physical activity, and emotional support, genuine change arises from active involvement. This empowerment is a key aspect of community engagement in health and well-being.

Ion's journey, a testament to the power of community ,vividly illustrates this. Initially hesitant, Ion found meaningful change through personal efforts and the supportive environment fostered by his heart health association. After his diagnosis of high cholesterol and early heart disease, he realized that maintaining his health required more than just medication. Encouraged by a friend, he reluctantly joined a community heart health program – what he thought would be a passive experience turned into a life-changing transformation, mainly due to the collective support of his community.

Through group discussions, shared meals, and structured physical activities, Ion understood that healing wasn't just an individual pursuit but a shared responsibility. The more he engaged with his community, the more he benefited. He found a deep sense of belonging in the stories of others, accountability in his friendships, and inspiration to adopt a healthier lifestyle. Over time, he improved his diet, became more active, and, most importantly, built meaningful connections that kept him committed to his health journey.

Community engagement - such as volunteering, local health advocacy, or building robust social connections – is consistently linked to better health outcomes. People who actively participate in their communities experience lower rates of chronic inflammation, improved mental health, and higher overall resilience. This reciprocity is crucial: giving back doesn't just uplift others; it significantly enhances one's health and emotional satisfaction, making community engagement a powerful tool for individual health improvement.

12.1 Building Healthy Communities

A robust, health-conscious community supports wellness by addressing several key elements:

Access to Nutritious Foods: Initiatives like community gardens, farmers' markets, and food cooperatives offer fresh, anti-inflammatory food options, reducing reliance on processed alternatives.

Opportunities for Physical Activity: Safe parks, walking trails, and community fitness programs encourage regular physical activity, promoting overall health and reducing sedentary lifestyles.

Health Education and Awareness: Workshops, public health campaigns, and community events educate residents about disease prevention and holistic health practices.

Emotional and Social Support: Strong networks of friends, neighbors, and support groups alleviate stress, cultivate belonging, and directly improve health outcomes.

Ion's experience demonstrates how these elements interplay effectively. Engaging with his community provided emotional reinforcement and practical guidance, transforming his health journey into a shared, uplifting experience.

12.2 Social Networks in Healing

Just as chronic inflammation is fuelled by isolation and unhealthy lifestyle choices, healing can be significantly enhanced through supportive social networks. Research confirms that individuals recovering from illnesses or managing chronic conditions improve faster and more sustainably when they have active support systems.

Peer Support Groups: Provide emotional strength and shared experiences for individuals dealing with chronic health issues, mental health challenges, or weight management.

Cultural and Faith-Based Support Systems: Many communities leverage shared meals, group wellness activities, and spiritual connections to enhance overall well-being.

Local Health Advocates and Mentors: Professionals like community health coaches and wellness leaders offer personalized guidance, helping individuals make informed decisions and sustainable lifestyle changes.

Ion's progress wasn't solitary but buoyed by his support group's collective wisdom and encouragement. His journey underlines the profound impact social networks can have in fostering sustainable, lifelong health transformations.

12.3 Taking an Active Role in Community Health

You Get Out What You Put In

Like any aspect of life, health is deeply influenced by effort and participation. The more we invest in our well-being and the well-being of our community, the greater the returns in terms of health, happiness, and longevity. A supportive community thrives when individuals actively contribute to its strength, just as personal health flourishes when we make consistent, intentional choices.

When people engage in community health initiatives – whether by participating in wellness programs, advocating for better resources, or simply fostering strong social connections - the benefits extend beyond the individual. Studies show that individuals who give back to their communities experience improved mental and physical health outcomes, reinforcing that healing is reciprocal. Healthcare professionals are crucial in these initiatives, providing guidance, support, and expertise.

On an individual level, investing in community health creates a ripple effect. When we commit to healthier habits, such as eating whole foods, staying active, and managing stress, we inspire and influence those around us. By setting an example, we contribute to a collective culture of well-being. Likewise, when communities invest in accessible healthcare, public spaces for movement, and mental health resources, individuals have a greater chance of thriving.

Ultimately, what we put into our health – personally and collectively – determines what we get in return. By actively engaging in our communities and prioritizing wellness, we build a strong foundation for better health for ourselves and future generations.

12.4 Global Engagement: A Collective Responsibility for Better Health

The Broader Impact of Global Health Initiatives

While family and community play foundational roles in shaping health, global factors also significantly influence well-being. Policies, economic systems, and international health initiatives impact food availability, medical access, and environmental conditions. Recognizing how global engagement affects personal health allows individuals to become informed advocates for a healthier world.

International efforts to combat chronic disease, malnutrition, and environmental pollution demonstrate that health is interconnected across borders. For example, the rise in chronic inflammation-related diseases is not confined to a single country – it is a global challenge requiring coordinated solutions. Climate change affects food security, international trade influences dietary habits, and medical accessibility varies dramatically worldwide. Addressing these disparities requires awareness and action at multiple levels.

The Role of Governments and Organizations in Public Health

Directly Impacts Health

Governments and international organizations shape public health through policies influencing food production, healthcare access, and environmental safety. Some key areas where global engagement directly impacts health include:

Food Policy and Nutrition Standards: International regulations determine the safety and quality of what we eat, impacting diet-related disease rates.

Environmental Health Protections: Air and water quality standards, pollution control, and climate change policies influence long-term health outcomes.

Access to Healthcare: Global health initiatives provide vaccines, medications, and preventive care in underserved regions, reducing disease   burdens worldwide.

The Hidden Contributors to Global Health Disparities
Disparities Hurt Everyone

Just as hidden contributors fuel chronic inflammation at the individual level, systemic factors silently shape global health disparities. These include:

Economic Inequality: Socioeconomic status affects healthcare access, quality nutrition, and disease prevention resources.

Food Industry Practices: The spread of ultra-processed foods contributes to rising obesity, diabetes, and heart disease rates worldwide.

Pharmaceutical and Medical Industry Influence: While medications save lives, an over-reliance on pharmaceuticals instead of preventive care has created unintended public health challenges.

12.5 Becoming an Active Participant in Global Health

Small Actions, Big Impact

Individuals can meaningfully contribute to global health, even without direct involvement in policy-making. Small actions that raise awareness, support ethical consumer choices, and promote health equity make a difference. Some steps include:

Advocate for Policy Change: Support initiatives promoting better food labeling, transparency in healthcare, and climate-friendly policies.

Support Ethical and Sustainable Practices: Choose food and products from companies prioritizing health and environmental responsibility.

Educate and Share Knowledge: Raising awareness about global health issues fosters informed decision-making at all levels of society.

A Shared Future: Health as a Global Priority

The health of individuals, communities, and nations is deeply interconnected. Acknowledging this, we move beyond isolated efforts and embrace a collective responsibility for well-being. True healing requires a shift in mindset – from viewing health as a personal issue to recognizing it as a shared commitment that transcends borders. When we invest in global health, we invest in a healthier, more sustainable future for all.

12.6 Conclusion: Bringing It All Together

A Collective Commitment to Health

Throughout this chapter, we have explored the interconnected nature of health- how healing extends beyond the individual to families, communities, and global systems. True well-being is not achieved in isolation; it is cultivated through relationships, shared values, and societal structures that support long-term health.

Healing together requires a shift in perspective. Instead of seeing health as a personal challenge, we must recognize it as a collective commitment. By fostering strong family connections, actively engaging in community initiatives, and advocating for global health equity, we contribute to a movement where well-being is accessible to all.

12.7 Small Actions, Big Impact

The Power of Health Literacy

A key component of collective well-being is health literacy – the ability to access, understand, and apply health-related information. When empowered with knowledge, individuals make informed choices that benefit themselves and their communities.

Breaking Down Misinformation: In a world of rapidly spreading information, distinguishing between credible health advice and misleading claims is crucial for making sound health decisions.

Building Confidence in Health Choices: Understanding nutrition, mental well-being, and preventive care enables individuals to take control of their health rather than relying solely on medical interventions.

Creating a Culture of Shared Knowledge: Families and communities prioritizing open health discussions foster environments where informed decisions become the norm.

Investing in health literacy strengthens individuals and communities, paving the way for better health outcomes and more effective public health initiatives.

12.8 The Ripple Effect of Conscious Choices

The Power of Conscious Decisions

Change does not require massive overhauls; it begins with small, intentional actions. When individuals make conscious decisions – choosing whole foods, prioritizing movement, supporting ethical businesses, or simply connecting with loved ones – these choices ripple outward, influencing families and communities.

Each decision we make carries weight. Changing to whole foods, walking more, or prioritizing time with loved ones – can spark momentum beyond the individual. When we model healthy behaviors, others take notice. A friend inspired by your dietary shift may start making more nutritious choices, a family member motivated by your daily movement may incorporate exercise into their own routine, and an entire community can slowly transition toward a culture of wellness.

The ripple effect of conscious choices is powerful. For example, one family committing to eating home-cooked meals together may improve their health and inspire extended family and friends to do the same. Likewise, businesses prioritizing ethical, sustainable sourcing contribute to healthier food systems, influencing consumer habits and industry standards.

Communities thrive when members invest in them. The more we contribute to the collective well-being, the more we strengthen our health in return. Each conversation, every shared meal, and every act of service plays a role in shaping a healthier society. Volunteering at a local wellness initiative, supporting a farmer's market, or advocating for more nutritious school lunches are all small yet significant actions that build healthier environments for everyone.

True health transformation begins with individual choices, but its real impact is seen in the communities we nurture. Whether promoting mental well-being, supporting ethical businesses, or engaging in shared wellness practices, every effort contributes to a broader movement toward sustainable, collective health.

12.9 The Path Forward

As we close this book, let this be a reminder that your health is deeply connected to the world around you. By nurturing your well-being and supporting the health of others, you become part of a larger movement toward healing. The journey does not end here – it continues with every choice, every action, and every connection you cultivate.

A year later, Ion had transformed the way he lived. He wasn't just healthier – he was thriving. His experience taught him that healing isn't just about personal willpower but about the people we surround ourselves with. Prevention is better than cure. So, Ion volunteered with other parents to help with health literacy and designing school meals.

In this chapter, we explored how family, community, and global engagement shape our health and how fostering supportive environments can help us all lead healthier, more fulfilling lives.

Healing together is not just an ideal - it is a necessity. And it starts with you. The best time to take action is now.

Your Healing Reflection:

- How could engaging with digital communities, local groups, or global initiatives strengthen your healing journey?

- What first step could you take to connect?

Please complete the 'I will ...' statement on page 5.

CONCLUSION

A Collective Commitment to Health

Throughout this book, we have explored the interconnected nature of health - how healing extends beyond the individual to families, communities, and global systems. True well-being is not achieved in isolation; it is cultivated through relationships, shared values, and societal structures that support long-term health.

Healing together requires a shift in perspective. Instead of seeing health as a personal challenge, we must recognize it as a collective commitment. By fostering strong family connections, actively engaging in community initiatives, and advocating for global health equity, we contribute to a movement where well-being is accessible to all.

The Power of Health Literacy

A key component of collective well-being is health literacy – the ability to access, understand, and apply health-related information. When empowered with knowledge, individuals make informed choices that benefit themselves and their communities.

- Breaking Down Misinformation: In a world of rapidly spreading information, distinguishing between credible health advice and misleading claims is crucial for making sound health decisions.

- Building Confidence in Health Choices: Understanding nutrition, mental well-being, and preventive care enables individuals to take control of their health rather than relying solely on medical interventions.

- Creating a Culture of Shared Knowledge: Families and communities prioritizing open health discussions foster environments where informed decisions become the norm.

Investing in health literacy strengthens individuals and communities alike, paving the way for better health outcomes and more effective public health initiatives.

The Path Forward

I know first hand however whelming it can feel to take control of your health, especially in a world that often makes it harder rather than easier. There were moments when I faced uncertainty, struggled to regain my strength, and wondered if lasting change was possible. But I also know the power of persistence, informed choices, and the support of a strong community. Healing is not about perfection – it is about progress, and every small step makes a difference.

A Stronger Kind of Health

True health is not just about physical strength or stamina. You can run marathons, lift heavy weights, or maintain a busy lifestyle – yet still be vulnerable if your mental and immunological health are overlooked.

Real wellness is a deeper kind of fitness:

- Physical strength to move and thrive

- Mental resilience to weather life's storms

- Immune vitality to protect, heal, and renew

This is the new foundation we must build - not just looking healthy, but being truly resilient from the inside out.

As you move forward, think beyond fitness.

Nurture your mind. Strengthen your immune system. Care for your body with intention and compassion.

Healing is not about chasing perfection. It's about creating balance, restoring vitality, and honoring the incredible body

Your Next Steps – Start Today

Real change doesn't come from grand gestures or overnight transformations. It comes from the little things – the everyday decisions that build momentum over time.

Swap one processed meal for a nutrient-dense option. Keep it simple – choose real, whole foods over packaged alternatives.

Move your body in a way that feels good. A short walk, stretching, or even standing more throughout the day – it all counts.

Prioritize sleep and recovery. Start with one habit -reduce screen time before bed, create a wind-down routine, or simply go to bed 30 minutes earlier.

Share what you've learned. Health isn't just personal; it's communal. When you share knowledge, you empower others.

Progress matters more than perfection. There will be days when you feel strong and motivated and others when old habits creep in. That's okay. The key is to keep going, to be patient with yourself, and to remember that every step forward – no matter how small – makes a difference.

You're Not Alone in This

Your journey is not one you have to navigate alone. There is a growing movement – people just like you – choosing prevention over prescriptions, reclaiming their health, and redefining what's possible.

Your choices don't just impact you – they ripple out to your family, your community, and future generations.

You become part of the solution when you choose to nourish your body, move with intention, and challenge the norms that have led to an epidemic of chronic disease. And that solution grows stronger when shared.

Stay Connected – Be Part of the Change

I am truly grateful that you've taken this journey with me. Your health matters. Your story matters. And your commitment to change is more powerful than you realize.

If you have questions, need support, or simply want to share your progress, I'd love to hear from you: *hemant.AIGuide@selfcarenation.co.uk*

But beyond that, I invite you to be part of something greater – a collective movement of individuals who are challenging outdated health narratives and proving that well-being is within our control.

Join the conversation. Share your experiences. Learn from others. Inspire and be inspired. Because when we come together, our collective impact is immeasurable. And, you already have everything you need to create lasting change.

So, take that first step. You've got this.

A Final Thought

As we close this book, let this be a reminder: your health is deeply connected to the world around you. By nurturing your well-being and supporting the health of others, you become part of a larger movement toward healing. The journey does not end here – it continues with every choice, every action, and every connection you cultivate.

Healing together is not just an ideal – it is a necessity. And it starts with you.

Your Healing Reflection:

- Reflecting on everything you have learned, what vision do you now hold for your healthiest, most vibrant future?

- What first commitment will you make today towards that vision?

Please review the 'I will …' statements on page 5 and <u>convert information in this book into YOUR transformation.</u>

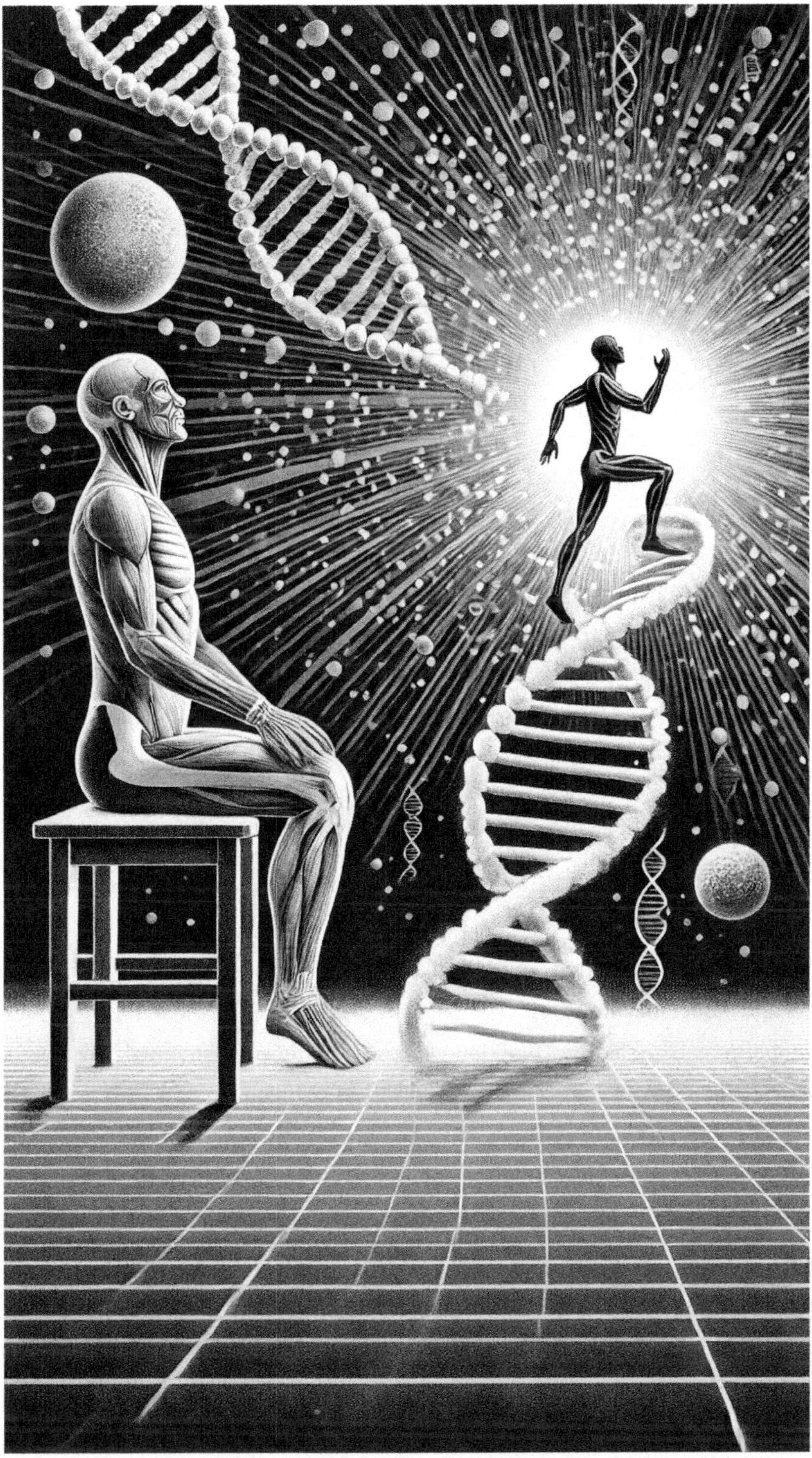

GLOSSARY AND REFERENCES

Glossary

A

Acute Inflammation – The body's short-term reaction to injury or infection, causing redness, swelling, heat, and pain to aid healing.

Aerobic Exercise – Any physical activity that raises the heart rate and improves oxygen use, like walking, cycling, or swimming.

Amyloid Plaques – Protein clumps in the brain linked to Alzheimer's disease, which disrupt nerve function.

Anti-Inflammatory Diet – Eating whole, unprocessed foods rich in vitamins and antioxidants while avoiding processed foods that trigger inflammation.

Antioxidants – Compounds in foods like berries and nuts that protect cells from damage and reduce inflammation.

Autoimmune Disorder – A condition where the immune system mistakenly attacks the body, causing chronic inflammation and diseases like rheumatoid arthritis.

Ayurveda – An ancient Indian healing system that balances diet, herbs, and lifestyle for well-being.

B

Batch Cooking – Preparing meals in advance for easy and healthy eating throughout the week.

B Vitamins (B6, B12, Folate) – Essential nutrients that support brain function, energy production, and red blood cell formation.

Body Mass Index (BMI) – A measure comparing weight to height, often used to assess body fat but criticized for inaccuracy.

C

Capsaicin – The active compound in chili peppers that reduces pain and inflammation.

Cardiovascular Disease (CVD) – A group of heart and blood vessel conditions, often caused by chronic inflammation.

Chronic Inflammation – A long-term immune response that damages tissues and increases the risk of diseases like diabetes and heart disease.

Circadian Rhythm – The body's internal clock that regulates sleep and daily biological functions.

Community Health Fair – A local event providing free health screenings, wellness workshops, and fitness activities.

Coenzyme Q10 (CoQ10) – A compound needed for energy production and heart health, often depleted by cholesterol-lowering medications.

Cortisol – The body's main stress hormone. Too much overtime can increase inflammation and lead to health problems.

C-Reactive Protein (CRP) – A protein the liver produces in response to inflammation; high levels indicate increased risk of disease.

Curcumin – The main active ingredient in turmeric, known for its anti-inflammatory effects.

Cytokines – Small proteins that help control the immune system, some of which cause inflammation while others reduce it.

D

Diuretics – Medications that help the body remove excess water but can also cause nutrient loss.

Digital Well-being – Using technology in a balanced way to support mental and physical health while avoiding screen overuse.

Drug-Induced Nutrient Deficiency (DIND) – When medications reduce the body's essential nutrients, increasing health risks.

E

Erythrocyte Sedimentation Rate (ESR) – A blood test that detects inflammation by measuring how fast red blood cells settle.

F

Fermentation – A natural process that increases good bacteria in foods like yogurt and kimchi, improving gut health.

Fiber – A nutrient found in plant-based foods that aids digestion, supports gut health, and helps regulate blood sugar.

Flavonoids – Plant-based antioxidants found in foods like dark chocolate and tea that help reduce inflammation.

Food Literacy – Understanding how food choices impact health, including meal planning and cooking skills.

G

Gut-Brain Connection – The link between gut health and brain function, affecting mood and mental well-being.

H

Hashtag Campaign – A social media trend where people post about a common goal, such as #30DaysOfHealth, to build a supportive community.

Healthy Fats – Beneficial fats from foods like olive oil and avocados that support heart and brain health.

High-Intensity Interval Training (HIIT) – Short bursts of intense exercise followed by rest, known for boosting fitness quickly.

HPA Axis – The system in the body that regulates stress and controls the release of cortisol.

Hydration – Drinking enough water to keep the body functioning properly and prevent dehydration.

I

Ikigai – A Japanese concept about finding purpose and meaning in daily life, linked to well-being and longevity.

Inflammaging – The slow build up of low-level inflammation that contributes to aging and chronic diseases.

Inflammatory Cytokines – Proteins that promote inflammation, often increasing with poor sleep or stress.

Insulin Resistance – When the body stops responding well to insulin, leading to high blood sugar and diabetes risk.

Insulin Sensitivity – How efficiently the body uses insulin to keep blood sugar levels stable.

M

Macronutrients – The three main nutrients the body needs: carbohydrates, proteins, and fats.

Meal Planning – Organizing meals ahead of time to support a balanced diet and healthy eating habits.

Mediterranean Diet – A way of eating rich in vegetables, fish, and olive oil, known for its anti-inflammatory benefits.

Microbiome – The community of trillions of microbes in the gut that play a role in digestion and immunity.

Mindful Eating – Eating with awareness, focusing on flavors and hunger cues to improve digestion and satisfaction.

Mindset Shift – A change in thinking that helps people take control of their health and make better choices.

Mitochondrial Function – How the body's cells produce energy, which is essential for overall health.

Myokines – Proteins released by muscles during exercise that help reduce inflammation.

O

Omega-3 Fatty Acids – Healthy fats found in fish, walnuts, and flaxseeds that help reduce inflammation.

Oxidative Stress – A harmful process where too many free radicals damage cells, contributing to aging and disease.

P

Pedometer – A device or app that counts steps and tracks physical activity.

Peer-Reviewed Study – Research that has been checked by experts to ensure it meets scientific standards.

Phytonutrients – Natural compounds in plants that help protect against diseases and inflammation.

Piperine – A compound in black pepper that helps the body absorb nutrients like curcumin from turmeric.

Polyphenols – Plant-based compounds that act as anti-oxidants and support overall health.

Processed Foods – Foods that have been altered from their natural state, often containing unhealthy additives.

Probiotics – Good bacteria found in foods like yogurt and supplements that improve gut health.

Pro-Inflammatory Cytokines – Proteins that increase inflammation and contribute to chronic diseases.

Proton Pump Inhibitors (PPIs) – Medications that reduce stomach acid but can lead to nutrient deficiencies.

S

SMART Goals – A method for setting clear and realistic health goals.

Social Media Health Communities – Online groups where people share advice and experiences about health and wellness.

Statins – Cholesterol-lowering drugs that may reduce levels of CoQ10, affecting muscle health.

T

Traditional Chinese Medicine (TCM) – A holistic healing system using acupuncture, herbs, and movement practices like tai chi.

Turmeric (Curcumin) – A bright yellow spice known for reducing inflammation and improving joint health.

V to Z

Visceral Fat – Fat stored deep in the abdomen that releases harmful inflammatory chemicals.

Volunteerism in Public Health – Helping with health initiatives like nutrition programs and fitness challenges to improve community well-being.

Whole Foods – Natural, unprocessed foods like fruits, vegetables, and lean proteins.

Za'atar – A Middle Eastern spice blend known for its health benefits.

Zinc – A mineral that supports immunity and healing, sometimes depleted by medications.

References

To keep things breezy for the printers (and save some trees, probably), we've stashed a detailed bibliography of all the books and papers used in this book's research online. Check it out here: selfcarenation.co.uk/sources

Printed in Great Britain
by Amazon